GASTRIC SLEEVE COOKBOOK #2020

Easy, Cheap and Fast Bariatric-Friendly
Recipes to Enjoy After Weight Loss Surgery |
For Every Stage of Bariatric Surgery Recovery

Dr. Julia Greene

Text Copyright ©

Legal & Disclaimer

The information contained in this book and its contents is not designed to replace or take the place of any form of medical or professional advice; and is not meant to replace the need for independent medical, financial, legal or other professional advice or services, as may be required. The content and information in this book has been provided for educational and entertainment purposes only.

The content and information contained in this book has been compiled from sources deemed reliable, and it is accurate to the best of the Author's knowledge, information and belief. However, the Author cannot guarantee its accuracy and validity and cannot be held liable for any errors and/or omissions. Further, changes are periodically made to this book as and when needed. Where appropriate and/or necessary, you must consult a professional (including but not limited to your doctor, attorney, financial advisor or such other professional advisor) before using any of the suggested remedies, techniques, or information in this book.

Upon using the contents and information contained in this book, you agree to hold harmless the Author from and against any damages, costs, and expenses, including any legal fees potentially resulting from the application of any of the information provided by this book. This disclaimer applies to any loss, damages or injury caused by the use and application, whether directly or indirectly, of any advice or information presented, whether for breach of contract, tort, negligence, personal injury, criminal intent, or under any other cause of action.

You agree to accept all risks of using the information presented inside this book.

You agree that by continuing to read this book, where appropriate and/or necessary, you shall consult a professional (including but not limited to your doctor, attorney, or financial advisor or such other advisor as needed) before using any of the suggested remedies, techniques, or information in this book.

Table of Contents

Introduction

Are you struggling with being obese? Have you tried all means to lose your weight without success? Are you planning to have a gastric sleeve surgery? Are you wondering how you can prepare for a gastric sleeve surgery?

This guide is going to offer you an overview of what exactly a Gastric Sleeve is and what you can expect before, during, and after this procedure. If this is a journey you have chosen to take with the goal towards a healthier quality of living, then this is the book written to assist you as you work towards your goals.

Gastric sleeve surgery is so beneficial for any person who is struggling to cut the weight and they have tried all other methods to no success. It is safe for most people. Try it today and you will be glad you chose to do it!

Happy reading!

Chapter 1: Sleeve Gastrectomy

What is sleeve gastrectomy

Sleeve gastrectomy is a surgical procedure for weight-loss. It is a restrictive operation that makes your stomach smaller so that you will feel fuller more quickly and eat less food. This procedure involves the removal of more than half of your stomach. The reduction is performed surgically by removing a portion along the greater curvature of the stomach. After your surgery, only a vertical tube about the size of a banana is left. The surgery has become a popular choice for people looking for extreme weight loss options.

This surgery should be considered as a tool for weight loss rather than a quick fix, because the patient will need to eat a healthy diet and exercise following the surgery. The gastric sleeve surgery is a simple medical procedure that removes parts of the stomach in order to lose weight. Not only will the surgery actually shrink your stomach and physically reduce the amount of food you can eat, it will change hormonal signals between the stomach, brain and the liver. In simple terms, your appetite and the need for food will be reduced. It is not cosmetic surgery where fat is removed. Only part of the stomach is removed.

Gastric sleeve and bariatric surgery

The method, known as a stomach or bariatric bypass operation, is the most commonly used procedure in the United States for surgery as a means of weight loss. Like the Gastric Sleeve procedure, in many instances, bypass surgery is irreversible. The surgery itself with a bypass requires a slight increase in the amount of time to perform. The Gastric Sleeve takes approximately an hour while the Bypass requires about 1.5 hours. Both surgeries require two to three days in hospital post-surgery (barring no complications arise), and a 2-4 week recovery period.

With the Bypass procedure, a surgeon may opt to use laparoscopy, similar to the Gastric Sleeve procedure, or they may make one 10-12 inch incision in the abdomen. The stomach itself is assessed, and a pouch is built along the top. The pouch area is defined by the insertion of surgical staples. This pocket will eventually be capable of holding up to one cup of food. An average stomach can hold up to 6 cups of food.

The surgeon then must attach the small intestine to this 'new' stomach which requires the food to move to the mid-section of small intestine, untouching the rest of the stomach and its connection to the upper areas. They then must join the upper small intestine to its mid-section, allowing for the flow of digestive fluids from the lower stomach to flow down from the upper small intestine into the mid-section of the intestine. The incision will then be closed by staples or stitches.

What is the use of performing sleeve gastrectomy

Less complicated than the other types of surgery

Gastric bypass is a complex surgery and takes an average of 4 hours to perform. There is a shorter variation of a gastric bypass surgery, but it's considered very difficult. The duodenal switch surgery is the most complicated because it involves a lot of rearranging. Since it's done in two parts, it can take up to three hours. Lap-band surgery is relatively short at one to two hours and isn't complicated for experienced doctors, but the gastric sleeve surgery only takes an hour and is considered the least challenging.

Doesn't trigger dumping syndrome

When you get parts of your stomach removed, dumping syndrome often results. This happens when sugar moves from your stomach to your small bowel too quickly. You will experience cramps, diarrhea, vomiting, dizziness, and other symptoms 10-30 minutes after eating. Dumping syndrome is especially common after eating meals high in sucrose or fructose. Gastric sleeve patients rarely get this, while it's commonly-associated with gastric bypass surgery.

Results in significant weight loss

Following gastric sleeve surgery, patients lose about 60-70% of excess weight in just a year. With exercise and proper eating, patients can lose even more weight in the coming years. Five years after surgery, on average, patients keep off over half of their extra weight. If you are diligent about diet, exercise, and doctor follow-ups, you can keep off all of it.

Can improve obesity-related diseases

When patients are sure to follow-up with their doctors following surgery, it's very common to see improvement in conditions like diabetes, hypertension, asthma, and more. Some even become cured. The benefits of maintaining a healthy weight cannot be overstated.

Less follow-up and risk of complications than other surgeries

For many, the most significant benefit of the gastric sleeve is less need for regular check-ups and less complications. Both gastric bypass and duodenal switch surgeries reduce the body's ability to absorb nutrition's, so blood tests are required for the rest of your life to prevent malnutrition. Tests are still necessary following gastric sleeve, but the follow-up isn't as intense because gastric sleeve surgery does not inhibit nutrition absorption.

Also, because both bypass and duodenal switch surgeries are more complicated, your risk for issues like pain, bloating, digestion problems, and more increases. As for lap-band surgery, regular adjustments to the band are required, while the presence of a foreign object in the body (the silicone band itself) can cause issues.

When can a patient opt for sleeve gastrectomy

The surgical option can apply to patients, who have tried all weight loss options such as exercise and diet control. Further, the following are also the conditions considered for sleeve gastrectomy

- The patient must be in extreme obese stage.

- The body mass index (BMI) should be more than 40 or higher.

- Some patients with a BMI of 35-39.9 and suffering from type 2 diabetes, other weight-related health issues, chronic sleep apnea, or high blood pressure.

- Sometimes the surgery also recommended for patients with a BMI of 30-34 but suffering from acute health issues due to obese.

Different types of bariatric surgery

Laparoscopic Adjustable Gastric Banding

A silicone elastic ring is placed surgically around the upper part of the stomach. The ring is then inflated with saline solution to tighten the opening from the upper abdomen to the lower belly so that the band decreases hunger and makes the patient eat less and still feel satisfied.

Sleeve Gastrectomy

In this process, 75 percent of stomach removed vertically, leaving a sleeve type portion for receiving food. During the dissection process, a considerable part of the stomach that produces ghrelin hormone, which is responsible for hunger feeling also get removed. The remaining portion will be producing less amount of hunger hormone; hence, the patient will feel less hunger.

As the nerves to the stomach and the valve leading from the stomach to the small intestine remain unchanged, this procedure preserves the functions of the stomach yet considerably reduces the volume. The small intestine remains unaffected.

Roux-En-y Gastric Bypass

This procedure splits the stomach into two sections surgically. The small upper part of the stomach surgically linked to the esophagus, which continues to receive food as usual, while the lower portion tinkered to dissociate from the food. The small intestine receives food directly from the newly created small stomach.

Duodenal Switch

Duodenal switch has two phases. In stage 1, the surgeon first performs a vertical sleeve gastrectomy procedure. After 12-18 months of the first surgery, the surgeon performs biliopancreatic diversion with duodenal switch. This process connects the remaining part of the stomach to the lower portion of the small intestine, causing significant malabsorption of calories and nutrients.

Revisional Surgery

Revisional procedures supplements and correct can maximizes the effectiveness of past surgery.

Preparations for gastric sleeve bariatric surgery

If you are planning for the bariatric surgery, doing a physical checkup will make sure whether the body is healthy to prepare for the procedure. But physical health is not the only requirement; a sound emotional state is also vital for a successful surgery and weight loss to follow.

Lifestyle Alterations:

You have to keep in mind that the real treatment doesn't begin or end with the gastric sleeve, and that is why it is critical for patients to start making changes before the surgery. Consult with your medical care team to get the right guidelines on lifestyle and behavioral alterations during the preparation of the surgery, which can even take months or up to a year.

During the time of preparation, the surgeon will devise the right diet plan by considering the age, health conditions, weight, and other characteristics of patients. Adopting healthy life habits and lifestyle changes increase the chance of losing more weight after the sleeve gastrostomy.

Confront a Food Addiction

If you are a food addict, then ensure that you address it before surgery. Having a small stomach trough bariatric surgery is not going to make things perfect; you need to control your eating patterns and emotional needs. These days, many people use food to battle daily stress.

But this is not the best way to manage our problem and can create further issues down the road. You have to be at a point where you have to recognize and confront any food addiction to change and feel better. Focus on your long-term goals, and learn to manage food to maintain your weight loss goals. Make sure that your food intake is sharply restricted primarily for the first few months. Also, eat food slowly so that it takes at least 20 minutes to finish your small meals. Stop grazing junk food to lose more pounds effectively

Start With Realistic Expectations

Do not expect yourself to wake up thin after bariatric surgery. In fact, you might weight more while leaving the hospital due to the accumulated fluid. Remember that the surgery is not an immediate answer to weight loss, but it is an internal tool in the form of a smaller stomach which helps you on your weight loss journey in the future.

It takes another six months to lose half of your excess weight. After that, it might take another year to reach your weight loss goal. Understand that your weight loss journey will take some time and of course, a lot of effort. Having a well-designed idea of the whole process will help you stay on track.

Pros and cons of sleeve gastrectomy

Pros

Less complicated than the other types of surgery

Gastric bypass is a complex surgery and takes an average of 4 hours to perform. There is a shorter variation of a gastric bypass surgery, but it's considered very difficult. The duodenal switch surgery is the most complicated because it involves a lot of rearranging. Since it's done in two parts, it can take up to three hours. Lap-band surgery is relatively short at one to two hours and isn't complicated for experienced doctors, but the gastric sleeve surgery only takes an hour and is considered the least challenging.

Doesn't trigger dumping syndrome

When you get parts of your stomach removed, dumping syndrome often results. This happens when sugar moves from your stomach to your small bowel too quickly. You will experience cramps, diarrhea, vomiting, dizziness, and other symptoms 10-30 minutes after eating. Dumping syndrome is especially common after eating meals high in sucrose or fructose. Gastric sleeve patients rarely get this, while it's commonly-associated with gastric bypass surgery.

Results in significant weight loss

Following gastric sleeve surgery, patients lose about 60-70% of excess weight in just a year. With exercise and proper eating, patients can lose even more weight in the coming years. Five years after surgery, on average, patients keep off over half of their extra weight. If you are diligent about diet, exercise, and doctor follow-ups, you can keep off all of it.

Can improve obesity-related diseases

When patients are sure to follow-up with their doctors following surgery, it's very common to see improvement in conditions like diabetes, hypertension, asthma, and more. Some even become cured. The benefits of maintaining a healthy weight cannot be overstated.

Less follow-up and risk of complications than other surgeries

For many, the most significant benefit of the gastric sleeve is less need for regular check-ups and less complications. Both gastric bypass and duodenal switch surgeries reduce the body's ability to absorb nutrition's, so blood tests are required for the rest of your life to prevent malnutrition. Tests are still necessary following gastric sleeve, but the follow-up isn't as intense because gastric sleeve surgery does not inhibit nutrition absorption.

Also, because both bypass and duodenal switch surgeries are more complicated, your risk for issues like pain, bloating, digestion problems, and more increases. As for lap-band surgery, regular adjustments to the band are required, while the presence of a foreign object in the body (the silicone band itself) can cause issues.

Cons

Gallstones

Gallstones are one of the most reported complications after gastric sleeve surgery. Within two years, 23% of patients get gallbladder disease. Sometimes surgeons will even remove the gallbladder while performing the surgery. Symptoms of gallstones include pain in your upper back and abdomen, nausea, vomiting, indigestion, bloating, gas, and heartburn. If the pain can't be numbed by regular pain medication; you're vomiting; or you have chills, sweats, or a fever, you should go to the ER.

Staple line leaks

A week following surgery, surgeons are most worried about staple line leaks. They aren't common - about 2.4% are at risk - but they're very serious. Symptoms include an increased heart rate, trouble breathing, and a fever. If you experience any of these three, call your doctor. If it's been three days or less since your surgery, surgeons will go back in with a laparoscope and repair the leak. If it's been 8 days or longer, you most likely won't have to go through surgery. Other treatment such as stents and drainage are more common at this point.

Blood clots

A surgery is a type of injury - you are being cut into - and blood clots are always a risk with an injury. They also tend to occur when you don't move a lot after your injury, which will happen following surgery. Clots can be life-threatening, so getting attention quickly is vital. Symptoms include numbness, redness, swelling, pain, and paleness in your arm and legs.

Strictures

A stricture is when the opening to your stomach (the actual stomach, not your surgery scar opening) or to your intestines get inflamed or blocked. This prevents food from making its normal journey through the body. You might have a stricture if you feel nauseated, have trouble swallowing, you're vomiting, or you can't eat certain foods.

Wound site infection

After surgery, the areas where the surgeon made incision cuts can become infected. Infection is a risk that comes with every type of surgery. If your incision areas feel hot or look red, or you're experiencing a fever, faster heart rate, lightheadedness, or dizziness, you might have an infection.

Nausea

You'll most likely feel nauseated during the first months following surgery. You might even need to vomit. Your body is doing a lot of healing and then adjusting to different foods.

Body aches

If these become too painful and you want to take a painkiller, ask your doctor which type is best. Common ones like Aleve and ibuprofen are usually not recommended.

Weakness and fatigue

Again, your body just went through a major surgery, so it needs rest. You're also consuming much less food, so your energy levels will be low.

Constipation

This happens because you aren't eating enough fiber. Drinking more fluids, taking fiber supplements, and walking can help.

Diarrhea or gas

You've most likely eaten something that's triggered stomach distress. Identify what you've eaten recently and then avoid it in the future.

Feeling cold

As you lose weight, you might feel colder than before. This is because fat insulates your body, and as you lose it, you lose that insulation.

Acne or dry skin

Some patients experience skin changes following weight-loss surgery. A healthy diet and the proper vitamins can help, as well as cleansers and lotions.

Hair loss

Hair loss is actually very common and occurs in 50% of patients following surgery. It happens because you are losing weight so quickly. The right diet, protein, and vitamins should help. You can also find special shampoos and supplements like flax seed oil.

Yeast infection

Antibiotics, which you take to prevent infection, can cause a yeast infection. Also known as thrush, this condition can result in a white coating on your tongue, redness, or inflammation. Talk to your doctor.

Moodiness

Feeling emotional after weight-loss surgery is very common. You might experience fear, anxiety, depression, uncertainty, or even regret. You might also feel frustrated about your recovery. The best solution is to stay connected to supportive friends and family and find peer support groups.

Complications of gastric-sleeve surgeries include gallstones, staple line leaks, blood clots, strictures, and wound site infections. Side effects, which are more common and usually less serious, include nausea, body aches, constipation, fatigue, and moodiness.

Chapter 2: Gastric sleeve diet

How to do and how to start a gastric sleeve diet

A gastric sleeve diet is a diet that is followed strictly by a person who intends to or has had a gastric sleeve surgery. It enables one's body to heal and adjust to a stomach with a smaller size.

Dieting Before Surgery

Your doctor may recommend a different two-week diet than the one we're going to discuss here, but this diet should serve as a golden rule (if you will call it that) for all pre-weight loss surgery diets. Begin by increasing your protein consumption by eating more lean meats, and lower your carbohydrate consumption. This means avoiding bread, pasta and rice. Finally, you'll need to eliminate all sugary foods completely. Candy, juice, soda, cake, you name it.

- For breakfast, try consuming more protein shakes such as from a supplement store. The only thing to watch out for in these shakes is to make sure that there are no sugars in them. For lunch and dinner alike, focus on eating more vegetables and lean meats.

- You can eat snacks throughout the day, but only ones that are healthy and low in carbs. Examples of this clued veggies, berries, nuts, and salads. It's also important that you stay hydrated throughout the days, so drinking plenty of water is critically important. An added benefit of water is that it will control the hunger you feel. Plus, it's common knowledge that water is good for you.

- In the three days before surgery, you will have to adhere to a strict liquid diet and stop drinking all beverages that are carbonated and/or have caffeine in them. Clear liquids that you can drink include protein shakes (though less shakes than you were consuming before), water, popsicles (provided they are sugar free), Jell-O, and broth.

- All in all, if you can adhere to this kind of strict surgery, the size of your liver should drastically decrease in the weeks before your surgery and the risk of developing any potential complications during surgery will dramatically decrease.

Dieting After Surgery

- For the first week, you'll have to adhere to clear liquids only. Whereas before you spent two to three days with only clear liquids, you're now going to have to add seven days to that. Fortunately, the ghrelin hormone will be nearly eliminated at this point, so your desire to eat high amounts of 'normal foods' will be nearly eliminated as well. Foods you can eat during this time, provided they are all sugar free, include water, un-carbonated drinks, broth, decaf tea and coffee. Specific foods that you should avoid include carbonated drinks, sweet drinks, non-decaf caffeine, and sugar.

- For the second week after surgery, you'll still have to adhere a liquid diet, but with less limitations than the clear liquid diet. For this week, you'll want to add more proteins to the mix. Examples of foods that you can eat during this time include protein powders mixed with liquid, sugar free ice cream, oatmeal, sugarless juices, creamy soups, nonfat yogurts, soupy noodles, and sugar free pudding. While this diet definitely has less limitations than before, you can't get too overconfident at this point and eat foods you shouldn't be eating.

- Good news! For the third week after surgery, you'll be able to add some real foods to your diet instead of strictly liquids. However, you should still keep your intake of fats and sugars down if not avoiding them completely. For this week, focus on taking smaller bites and eating the individual bites more slowly, only trying one new food per meal (meaning you should not have two or more kinds of foods at the same meal), and continue to get plenty of protein. This is because you must give your body the time it needs to react to these 'new' foods; remember that's gone well over a month by now without the foods it is used to in taking and digesting. It will need more time to adjust fully.

- There are specific new foods that you can now add to your diet, as well as a few others that you should continue to avoid. New foods that you can add are protein shakes mixed with yogurt and non-fat milk, hummus, low fat cheese, mashed fruit, canned tuna or salmon, mayonnaise, steamed fish (as long as you chew well), scrambled eggs, soup, grounded beef, grounded chicken, soft cereals (tip: allow your cereal to sit in the milk to become soft), soft vegetables, soft cheese, almond milk, and coconut milk. None of these foods should be crunchy and you should remember to chew slowly with all of them.

- Foods that you should continue to avoid in the third week are sugars, pasta, rice, bread, fibrous vegetables, and smoothies with high sugar levels.

- For the fourth week, you can continue to introduce more real foods that you're accustomed to. Remember though, your stomach is still very sensitive, and you aren't yet at the point where you can eat anything you want however you want. You still have to eat slowly, eat soft foods whenever possible, and only introduce one new food per meal.

- During this time, you should continue consuming protein shakes, as they are one of your best sources of protein throughout this dieting process. You can introduce more fish, fruits, softened vegetables, chicken and beef. All of these foods should be as softened as much as possible and chewed thoroughly. You can also re-introduce potatoes to your diet (mashed, baked and sweetened alike) and cereal. You can also re-introduced caffeine products to your diet, but not to the point that it becomes a regular part of your diet. Be very discretionary as you add caffeine to your diet.

- For the fourth week, you should focus primarily on eating three small meals throughout the day and getting plenty of water. But as long as your surgeon approves it, you should also be able to add snacks to your diet at this point. Examples of snacks that you can add include fresh fruit, small portions of baked or sweetened potatoes, small portions of oatmeal, one egg, a small portion of baby carrots, or a small portion of crackers.

- Some foods you will have to continue to avoid. Most sodas, fried food, fibrous vegetables, candy and sugar, desserts, pasta, pizzas, whole milk, dairy in general, and nuts will all have to continue to be avoided in the fourth week of your diet.

- For the fifth week, your body will be able to tolerate more foods, but you could still feel an upset stomach at times. Continue to eat three small meals and remain fully hydrated throughout the day. Continue to take your prescribed medication and vitamins, and focus mainly on getting enough protein into your system (sixty grams at the least). Again, protein shakes are an excellent way to get plenty of protein in your system. You should also try to exercise more now, and your body should start to lose weight at a faster rate. Continue to adhere to a strict dieting plan, and when you do eat snacks, only eat from small portions.

What are the foods you have to eat for a gastric sleeve diet

After gastric sleeve surgery, individuals required to consume vitamin and mineral supplements throughout their life.

Multivitamin & Mineral:

The patient needs to take two adult multivitamin-mineral supplements per day, which include folic acid, copper, iron, selenium, thiamin, and zin. The preferred option is chewable multivitamin and mineral supplement, which has a minimum 18mg iron and 400mcg folic acid, zinc, and copper daily.

Vitamin b12:

Daily consume 350-500mg of vitamin B12, either liquid or tablet. Nasal spray or injection are also optional to overcome the B12 deficiencies weekly once or 1cc injection per month.

Vitamin b Complex With Thiamine:

Patients must take 75-100 mg per day

Calcium Citrate:

Per day a patient needs to consume 1,200 to 2,000mg of calcium citrate to offshoot the calcium deficiency. For increased absorption, take three doses of 600mg per day.

Vitamin d:

Consume 800 to 1,000 IU per day. A patient can consume 400 to 500 IU two times per day, along with a calcium supplement. In case you want to take Calcium and vitamin D supplement combination tablet make sure, it has the right combination.

Iron:

45-60mg elemental Fe per day, which can have from multivitamin and supplements. Iron must be taken along with Vitamin C, not along with Calcium. 500mg per day is the dose for Vitamin C.

Food and DrinksTo Avoid After Gastric Sleeve Surgery

Alcohol:

You shouldn't consume alcohol at least one year after your gastric sleeve surgery. Due to the massive amount of weight loss, your body is quite stressed. Alcohol is not healthy; it has zero nutritional value and will only cause problems for you. Since the space in the stomach reduced drastically, there won't be enough space for food. Also, the rate of alcohol absorption will be very high, and that can lead to heavy intoxication.

Food With No Calories:

After gastric sleeve surgery, you must avoid foods with no calories. Because you are left with a tiny portion of the stomach after the surgery. There won't be enough space to accommodate too much food, the way you used to have before the surgery. So, you must consume nutritional rich food. Too much food loaded with sugar can lead to dumping syndrome, which will be a reason for nausea, diarrhea, vomiting, etc.

Red Meat:

For the first six months, avoid eating red meat. Red meat contains a lot of fibers which makes it hard to get processed by your stomach. And even though this kind of meat is healthy, you should eat something lighter instead such as crab, lamb, fish or shrimp. While consuming meats, you must chew it properly. Avoid beef, pork, ham, and hot dogs.

Bread, Pasta, And Rice:

All these food items are of rich in starch and hence required water consumption along with it while consuming. Because of the high start content, it will form like a paste and can even block the new stomach. During the initial recouping stage, try to avoid these items and on the later stage limit its consumption.

Dry Foods:

The gastric sleeve does not encourage people to drink water along with food. Since the food storage area in the stomach is too small, and there will be only a limited area for digestion. If you drink water along with food, there are chances that the consumed food may get discharged

20

without any digestion process. So, since you are not supposed to drink water while consuming dry foods, it will be difficult for you to swallow. The recommended food pattern during the recouping stage is liquified foods, stick to the diet plan that is tolerable to your body after the surgery. Once your body starts to adjust to the new lifestyle, you can begin consuming dry foods in a limited quantity.

Caffeinated Drinks:

Caffeinated drinks are harmful to your body under normal circumstances; you can only imagine the harm they would do when your stomach is under so much pressure. The carbonization of these drinks causes bloating and gas and lead to dumping syndrome, which occurs when sugar moves too quickly from your stomach to the bowel. It can cause weakness, abdominal pain and discomfort, nausea, and severe diarrhea.

Fibrous Vegetables And Fruits:

It is essential to consume nutrient-rich fruits and vegetables after gastric sleeve. However, you need to avoid vegetables and fruits that are tough to digest. You must avoid broccoli, celery, cabbage, corn, asparagus, etc., during the early days of the post-operation diet plan.

Food with High Fats:

Consumption of a high-fat diet after surgery may develop nausea, and it is not wise to consume for meeting the weight loss objectives. Avoid all types of high-fat foods such as whole milk, sausages, butter, bacon, fat-rich cheese, etc. Consuming excess fat-food also may be a reason for dumping syndrome.

How to eat again after a surgery

The following tips will help you to eat again after a surgery;

- The first tip is to eat foods that have plenty of nutrients in them. Examples of foods that are include most fruits like apples and bananas, as well as fish. Other foods such as grains, pasta or bread are not filled with as many nutrients.

- The second tip is to be prepared to feel emotional over your change in diet. But as long as you receive plenty of support from those you are close with and make it your mission to stick to your regimen, things will be okay.

- The next tip is to not fall to the temptations of restaurants. Eating out is perfectly fine, but don't feel you are obligated to eat everything on your plate. You can also ask for mid or half sized portions.

- Finally, and this cannot be enunciated enough, stay hydrated every day! Take plenty of water wherever you go and drink plenty of it. The difference between staying hydrated and not being hydrated will be huge when it comes to losing weight.

How to control food cravings after gastric sleeve

Don't Skip Meals

If you skip an already planned snack or meal, you are putting yourself at risk of getting extreme hunger pangs later. With hunger comes craving and urge to eat unhealthy food. Give your body proper food before you lose control.

Resist Sweets

I know, resisting sweets doesn't come easy. Rather than depriving yourself until you crave, you can indulge in a little with small servings. If you crave for chocolate, have a small piece of dark chocolate. However, be careful to avoid processed sugar and candies as it comes with a lot of calories and fat content.

Divert Your Focus

When you crave for a particular food, divert your concentration on something other than food. Try doing things you like, indulge in another activity, read a book, or talk to a friend. Don't force yourself not to think about your craving as that will cause to stick on to that particular thing even more. Get your mind off from that and do something else; you can even go for a walk.

Remind Your Goals

This one is pretty difficult, I understand. Bariatric surgery is a big decision you have taken after going through a lot of research and understanding. You already know your goals, but sometimes you need to remember the things you already know. Have a look into an old picture of yours if it matches your weight loss goals or reminds yourself how far you have come. Ask yourself whether giving in to your temporary craving will help or hinder the process you have made till now.

Drink Water

Whenever you feel like craving strikes in, grab a glass of water to make sure that what you crave for is water and not just anything else. Sometimes, dehydration can cause cravings and leads to grazing and overeating. Heavily hydrated people often experience fewer cravings, and you feel better throughout the day.

Demonstrate Self Compassion

If you want to kick-start your weight loss journey at a faster pace, first you have to cut the mental fat-which leads to cutting off the waistline fat. When trying to improve lifestyle and diet, most people do find until some interference happen-like work pressure, family problems, relationship issues, or something else. In that scenario, you ensure that you keep the momentum to continue your journey.

You are indeed on a tough mission, and it's not okay to give up. But some people emphasize more on this and pressurize them hindering weight loss again due to stress. Some even go overboard by reducing portion too much, skipping meals and punishing their body by thinking that less food intake leads to weight loss.

Here are some tips and tricks to keep with your weight loss journey while developing a deep self-compassion.

Set Realistic Goals And Expectations

When setting realistic goals, you also have to include cheat days giving room for a slight indulgence. For many, goals are unrealistic and hard to stick with, which leads to mental stress when they are not able to follow it.

Get Help When Needed

It is common for people who undergo bariatric surgery to crave for mental support at any phase before or after the surgery. If you feel like you need help or counseling after the surgery, get this done or else it can even lead to mental stress and depression.

Navigating Fear

As you have done the weight loss surgery, you might be experiencing a sort of relief as you have made a significant step accounting to your weight loss journey. But along with relief, comes worry. Worry about whether bowel obstruction or dumping syndrome could happen or what if you don't get the weight off post-surgery.

All you have to do is to give yourself time to get used to your new body. Stay committed to your lifestyle changes, and if you hit a weight loss plateau, you can talk to your doctor. There are dietary changes and workout that can help you overcome the plateau. It is not easy, but never impossible.

How to and best ways to eat out

- Never go after foods that are difficult to swallow. Avoid foods such as bread, steak, and fibrous vegetables. Avoid any food that you had never tried at home.

- Don't succumb to temptations to order foods the way how everyone is doing. Remember, you are not in a position to consume a large portion of food. The surgery had confined the stomach size like a sleeve. Select healthy foods and order for small portions.

- Ask foods like dressing and sauces separately in a plate or serving bowl.

- Avoid French fries or any other fried items. You can go for salads or cooked vegetables that are easy to digest.

- Make sure the ingredients of the food, and it must be low sugar, low carbs, and low fat. Never order any fried foods, instead go for broiled, steamed, poached, air-fried, baked or grilled foods.

- If the ordered food is beyond your toleration level, then ask the bearer to reduce the quantity and keep it away from your table. In doing so, you won't be tempted to eat excess quantity.

- After gastric sleeve, your stomach can not take ice cream or pudding. Therefore, avoid it.

- Instead of heavy drinks and beverages, try some soft drinks such as red-wine or low-calorie beverages.

- Do not drink carbonated items.

- Order foods cooked without oil or butter.

- Limit the intake of dessert or appetizer. Go for it if you can share it with your friends.

Chapter 3: Foods and liquids

What foods and liquids a person can eat and drink in a gastric sleeve diet

Liquids

Vitamin water

Sugar free Jell-O

Water

Sugar free popsicles

Diluted apple juice

Ice chips

Herbal teas

Diluted cranberry juice

Diluted white grape juice

Beef broth

Chicken broth

Butternut soup

Tomato soup

Low-sugar canned fruit

Low or no-sugar smoothies

Foods

One protein shake a day

Low-fat cottage cheese

Softened, low or no-sugar cereals

Steamed or boiled vegetables

Soup

Scrambled eggs

Soft steamed fish

Canned fish

Mashed bananas and avocados

Chapter 4: Recipes

Breakfast

Cherry Avocado Smoothie

Prep time: 5 minutes

Serves: 3

Difficulty: Intermediate

Ingredients:

- ½ ripe avocado, chopped
- 1 cup fresh cherries
- 1 cup coconut water, sugar-free
- 1 whole lime

Instructions:

1. Peel the avocado and cut in half. Remove the pit and chop into bite-sized pieces. Reserve the rest in the refrigerator. Set aside.

2. Rinse the cherries under cold running water using a large colander. Cut each in half and remove the pits. Set aside.

3. Peel the lime and cut in half. Set aside.

4. Now, combine avocado, cherries, coconut water, and lime in a blender. Pulse to combine and transfer to a serving glass.

5. Add few ice cubes and refrigerate for 10 minutes before serving.

Nutritional Value Per Serving:

Net carbs 17 g

Sugar 3 g

Fiber 3.8 g

Calories 128

Fats 6.8 g

Guava Smoothie

Prep time: 5-7 minutes

Serves: 2

Difficulty: Beginners

Ingredients:

- 1 cup guava, seeds removed, chopped
- 1 cup baby spinach, finely chopped
- 1 banana, peeled and sliced
- 1 tsp fresh ginger, grated
- ½ medium-sized mango, peeled and chopped
- 2 cups water

Instructions:

1. Peel the guava and cut in half. Scoop out the seeds and wash it. Cut into small pieces and set aside.
2. Rinse the baby spinach thoroughly under cold running water. Drain well and torn into small pieces. Set aside.
3. Peel the banana and chop into small chunks. Set aside.
4. Peel the mango and cut into small pieces. Set aside.
5. Now, combine guava, baby spinach, banana, ginger, and mango in a juicer and process until well combined. Gradually add water and blend until all combined and creamy.
6. Transfer to a serving glass and refrigerate for 20 minutes before serving.
7. Enjoy!

Nutritional Value Per Serving:

Net carbs 39.1 g   Fats 1.4 g   Calories 166

Fiber 7.8 g   Sugar 2 g

Veggie Quiche Muffins

Prep time: 10 minutes

Cook time: 40 minutes

Serves: 12

Difficulty: Intermediate

Ingredients:

- ¾ cup shredded cheddar
- 1 cup green onion
- 1 cup chopped broccoli
- 1 cup diced tomatoes
- 2 cup milk
- 4 eggs
- 1 cup pancake mix
- 1 tsp. oregano
- ½ tsp. salt
- ½ tsp. pepper

Instructions:

1. Set oven to 375 degrees F, and lightly grease a 12-cup muffin tin with oil.
2. Sprinkle tomatoes, broccoli, onions and cheddar into muffin cups.
3. Combine remaining ingredients in a medium bowl, whisk to combine then pour evenly on top of veggies.
4. Set to bake in preheated oven for about 40 minutes or until golden brown.
5. Allow to cool slightly (about 5 minutes) then serve. Enjoy!

Nutritional Value Per Serving:

Net carbs 2.9 g

Fiber 4 g

Fats 3.2 g

Sugar 1 g

Calories 58.8

Steel Cut Oat Blueberry Pancakes

Prep time: 7 minutes

Cook time: 13 minutes

Serves: 4

Difficulty: Intermediate

Ingredients:

- 1½ cup water
- ½ cup oats
- 1/8 tsp. salt
- 1 cup flour
- ½ tsp. baking powder
- ½ tsp. baking soda
- 1 egg
- 1 cup milk
- ½ cup Greek yogurt
- 1 cup frozen blueberries
- ¾ cup agave nectar

Instructions:

1. Combine oats, salt, and water together in a medium saucepan, stir, and allow to come to a boil over high heat.

2. Set it to low and simmer for 10 mins, or until oats are tender. Set aside.

3. Combine all remaining ingredients, except agave nectar, in a medium bowl, then fold in oats.

4. Preheat griddle and lightly grease. Cook ¼ cup of batter at a time for about 3 minutes per side.

5. Garnish with agave.

Nutritional Value Per Serving:

Net carbs 46 g

Fiber 1 g

Fats 7 g

Sugar 2 g

Calories 257

Very Berry Muesli

Prep time: 6 hours

Serves: 2

Difficulty: Beginner

Ingredients:

- 1 cup oats
- 1 cup fruit flavored yogurt
- ½ cup milk
- 1/8 tsp. salt
- ½ cup dried raisins
- ½ cup chopped apple
- ½ cup frozen blueberries
- ¼ cup chopped walnuts

Instructions:

1. Combine yogurt, salt and oats together in a medium bowl, mix well, then cover the mixture tightly.
2. Place in the refrigerator to cool for 6 hours.
3. Add raisins, and apples the gently fold.
4. Top with walnuts and serve. Enjoy!

Nutritional Value Per Serving:

Net carbs 31.2 g

Fiber 4 g

Fats 4.3 g

Sugar 3 g

Calories 198

Strawberry & Mushroom Breakfast Sandwich

Prep time: 10 minutes

Serves: 4

Difficulty: Beginner

Ingredients:

- 8 oz. Cream cheese
- 1 tbsp. Honey
- 1 tbsp. grated Lemon zest
- 4 sliced Portobello Mushrooms
- 2 cup sliced Strawberries

Instructions:

1. Add honey, lemon zest and cheese to a food processor, and process until fully incorporated.
2. Use cheese mixture to spread on mushrooms as you would butter.
3. Top with strawberries. Enjoy!

Nutritional Value Per Serving:

Net carbs 6 g

Fiber 2 g

Fats 16 g

Sugar 2 g

Calories 180

Turkey Sausage and Mushroom Strata

Prep time: 10 minutes

Cook time: 8 minutes

Serves: 12

Difficulty: Expert

Ingredients:

- 8 oz. cubed ciabatta bread
- 12 oz. chopped turkey sausage
- 2 cup milk
- 4 oz. shredded cheddar
- 3 eggs
- 12 oz. egg substitute

- ½ cup chopped green onion
- 1 cup sliced mushroom
- ½ tsp. paprika
- ½ tsp. pepper
- 2 tbsps. grated parmesan cheese

Instructions:

1. Set oven to 400 degrees F. Lay bread cubes flat on a baking tray and set it to toast for about 8 min.

2. Meanwhile, add a skillet over medium heat with sausage and allow to cook while stirring, until fully brown and crumbled.

3. In a bowl, add pepper, parmesan cheese, egg substitute, salt, paprika, eggs, cheddar cheese and milk, then whisk to combine.

4. Add in remaining ingredients and toss well to incorporate. Transfer mixture to a large baking dish (preferably a 9x13-inch) then tightly cover and allow to rest in the refrigerator overnight.

5. Set oven to 350 degrees F, remove the cover from casserole dish and set to bake until fully cooked and golden brown.

6. Slice and serve.

Nutritional Value Per Serving:

Net carbs 9.2 g

Fiber 2 g

Fats 18 g

Sugar 6 g

Calories 185

Sweet Millet Congee

Prep time: 5 minutes

Cook time: 15 minutes

Serves: 4

Difficulty: Beginner

Ingredients:

- 1 cup millet
- 5 cup water
- 1 cup diced sweet potato
- 1 tsp. cinnamon
- 2 tbsps. stevia
- 1 diced apple
- ¼ cup honey

Instructions:

1. In a deep pot, add stevia, sweet potato, cinnamon, water and millet, then stir to combine.
2. Bring to boil over high heat, then reduce to a simmer on low for an hour or until water is fully absorbed and millet is cooked.
3. Stir in remaining ingredients and serve.

Nutritional Value Per Serving:

Net carbs 28.5 g

Fiber 1 g

Fats 1 g

Sugar 3 g

Calories 136

Summer Breakfast Quinoa Bowls V

Prep time: 5 minutes

Cook time: 20 minutes

Serves: 2

Difficulty: Intermediate

Ingredients:

- 1 sliced peach
- 1/3 cup quinoa
- 1 cup low fat milk
- ½ tsp. vanilla extract
- 2 tsps. natural stevia
- 12 raspberries
- 14 blueberries
- 2 tsps. honey

Instructions:

1. Add natural stevia, 2/3 cup milk and quinoa to a saucepan, and stir to combine.
2. Over medium high heat, bring to a boil then cover and reduce heat to a low simmer for a further 20 minutes (you should be able to fluff quinoa with a fork).
3. Grease and preheat grill to medium. Grill peach slices for about a minute per side. Set aside.
4. Heat remaining milk in the microwave and set aside.
5. Split cooked quinoa evenly between 2 serving bowls and top evenly with remaining ingredients. Enjoy!

Nutritional Value Per Serving:

Net carbs 36 g

Fiber 4 g

Fats 4 g

Sugar 3 g

Calories 180

Perfect Granola

Prep time: 10 minutes

Cook time: 30 minutes

Serves: 10

Difficulty: Intermediate

Ingredients:

- ¼ cup canola oil
- 4 tbsps. honey
- 1½ tsp. vanilla
- 6 cup old fashioned rolled oats
- 1 cup almond
- ½ cup shredded unsweetened coconut
- 2 cup bran flakes
- ¾ cup chopped walnuts
- 1 cup raisins
- Cooking spray

Instructions:

1. Prepare oven to preheat at 325 degrees F.
2. In a saucepan, cook oil and vanilla gently over low flame, occasionally stirring for roughly 5 mins.
3. Place all ingredients except raisins into a large bowl and combine.
4. Stir in honey and oil mixture slowly, ensuring all grains are properly coated.
5. Set a parchment paper on the baking tray or use cooking spray to grease lightly. Spread cereal evenly in the tray and bake for 25 mins, occasionally stirring to keep mixture from burning, or until very lightly browned.
6. When ready, remove cereal and put aside to cool.
7. Add raisins and mix well.

Nutritional Value Per Serving:

Net carbs 62 g

Fiber 2 g

Fats 21 g

Sugar 3 g

Calories 458

Lunch

Fresh Shrimp Spring Rolls

Prep time: 20 minutes

Serves: 12

Difficulty: Beginner

Ingredients:

- 12 sheets rice paper
- 12 bib lettuce
- 12 basil laves
- ¾ cup cilantro
- 1 cup shredded carrots
- ½ sliced cucumber
- 20 oz. cooked shrimp

Instructions:

1. Add all vegetables and shrimp to separate bowls.
2. Set a damp paper towel tower flat on work surface.
3. Quickly wet a sheet of rice papers under warm water and lay on paper towel.
4. Top with 1 of each vegetable and 4 pieces of shrimp, then roll in rice paper into a burrito – like roll.
5. Repeat until all vegetables and shrimp has been used up. Serve and enjoy.

Nutritional Value Per Serving:

Net carbs 7.4 g

Fiber 7 g

Fats 2.9 g

Sugar 7 g

Calories 67

Sunshine Wrap

Prep time: 30 minutes

Serves: 2

Difficulty: Intermediate

Ingredients:

- 8 oz. grilled chicken breast
- ½ cup diced celery
- 2/3 cup mandarin oranges
- ¼ cup minced onion
- 2 tbsps. mayonnaise

- 1 tsp. soy sauce
- ¼ tsp. garlic powder
- ¼ tsp. black pepper
- 1 whole wheat tortilla
- 4 lettuce leaves

Instructions:

1. Combine all ingredients, except tortilla and lettuce, in a large bowl and toss to evenly coat.
2. Lay tortillas on a flat surface and cut into quarters.
3. Top each quarter with a lettuce leaf and spoon chicken mixture into the middle of each.
4. Roll each tortilla into a cone and seal by slightly wetting the edge with water. Enjoy!

Nutritional Value Per Serving:

Net carbs 3 g

Fiber 2 g

Fats 21.1 g

Sugar 9 g

Calories 280.8

Sweet Roasted Beet & Arugula Tortilla Pizza V

Prep time: 10 minutes

Cook time: 10 minutes

Serves: 6

Difficulty: Expert

Ingredients:

- 2 chopped Beets
- 6 Corn Tortillas
- 1 cup Arugula
- ½ cup Goat cheese

- 1 cup Blackberries
- 2 tbsps. Honey
- 2 tbsps. Balsamic vinegar

Instructions:

1. Preheat oven to 350 F. Lay tortillas on a flat surface.

2. Top with beets, berries and goat cheese. Combine balsamic vinegar and honey together in a small bowl, and whisk to combine.

3. Drizzle the mixture over pizza and to bake for about 10 minutes, or until cheese has melted slightly and tortilla is crisp.

4. Garnish with arugula and serve.

Nutritional Value Per Servin:

Net carbs 42 g

Fiber 2 g

Fats 40 g

Sugar 5 g

Calories 286

Southwestern Black Bean Cakes with Guacamole

Prep time: 5 minutes

Cook time: 10 minutes

Serves: 4

Difficulty: Expert

Ingredients:

- 1 cup whole wheat bread crumbs
- 3 tbsps. chopped cilantro
- 2 garlic cloves
- 15 oz. black beans
- 7 oz. chipotle peppers in adobo sauce
- 1 tsp. ground cumin
- 1 large egg
- ½ diced avocado
- 1 tbsp. lime juice
- 1 tomato plum

Instructions:

1. Drain beans and add all ingredients, except avocado, lime juice and eggs, to a food processor and run until the mixture begins to pull away from the sides.

2. Transfer to a large bowl and add egg, then mix well.

3. Form into 4 even patties and cook on a preheated, greased grill over medium heat for about 10 minutes, flipping halfway through.

4. Add avocado and lime juice in a small bowl, then stir and mash together using a fork.

5. Season to taste then serve with bean cakes.

Nutritional Value Per Serving:

Net carbs 25 g

Fiber 10 g

Fats 7 g

Sugar 3 g

Calories 178

Veggie Quesadillas with Cilantro Yogurt Dip

Prep time: 4 minutes

Cook time: 5 minutes

Serves: 3

Difficulty: Intermediate

Ingredients:

- 1 cup black beans
- 2 tbsps. chopped cilantro
- ½ chopped bell pepper
- ½ cup corn kernels
- 1 cup shredded cheese
- 6 corn tortillas
- 1 shredded carrot

Instructions:

1. Set skillet to preheat on low heat. Lay 3 tortillas on a flat surface.

2. Top evenly with peppers, carrots, cilantro, beans, corn and cheese over the tortillas, covering each with another tortilla, maximum.

3. Add quesadilla to preheated skillet. Cook until the cheese melts and tortilla is a nice golden brown (about 2 min).

4. Flip quesadilla and cook for about a minute or until golden.

5. Mix well. Slice each quesadilla into 4 even wedges and serve with dip. Enjoy!

Nutritional Value Per Serving:

Net carbs 46 g

Fiber 6 g

Fats 8 g

Sugar 8 g

Calories 344

Mayo-less Tuna Salad

Prep time: 5 minutes

Serves: 2

Difficulty: Beginner

Ingredients:

- 5 oz. tuna

- 1 tbsp. olive oil

- 1 tbsp. red wine vinegar

- ¼ cup chopped green onion

- 2 cup arugula

- 1 cup cooked pasta

- 1 tbsp. parmesan cheese

- Black pepper

Instructions:

1. Combine all ingredients into a medium bowl. Split mixture between two plates. Serve, and enjoy.

Nutritional Value Per Serving:

Net carbs 20.3 g

Fiber 4 g

Fats 6.2 g

Sugar 2 g

Calories 213.2

46

Southwest Style Zucchini Rice Bowl

Prep time: 5 minutes

Cook time: 4 minutes

Serves: 2

Difficulty: Intermediate

Ingredients:

- 1 tbsp. vegetable oil
- 1 cup chopped vegetables
- 1 cup chopped chicken breast
- 1 cup cooked zucchini rice
- 4 tbsps. salsa
- 2 tbsps. shredded cheddar cheese
- 2 tbsps. sour cream

Instructions:

2. Set a skillet with oil to heat up over medium heat.

3. Add chopped vegetables and allow to cook, stirring until vegetables become fork tender.

4. Add chicken and zucchini rice. Cook while stirring, until fully heated through.

5. Split between 2 serving bowls and garnish with remaining ingredients. Serve and enjoy!

Nutritional Value Per Serving:

Net carbs 18 g

Fiber 5 g

Fats 8.2 g

Sugar 1 g

Calories 168

Pesto & Mozzarella Stuffed Portobello Mushroom Caps

Prep time: 5 minutes

Cook time: 15 minutes

Serves: 2

Difficulty: Beginner

Ingredients:

- 2 portobello mushrooms
- 1 diced Roma tomato
- 2 tbsps. pesto
- ¼ cup sshredded mozzarella cheese

Instructions:

1. Spoon pesto evenly into mushroom caps, then top with remaining ingredients.
2. Bake at 400 degrees F for about 15 minutes. Enjoy!

Nutritional Value Per Serving:

Net carbs 7.5 g

Fiber 2 g

Fats 5.4 g

Sugar 2 g

Calories 112

Cold Tomato Couscous

Prep time: 15 minutes

Cook time: 10 minutes

Serves: 4

Difficulty: Expert

Ingredients:

- 5 oz couscous
- 3 tbsp tomato sauce
- 3 tbsp lemon juice
- 1 small-sized onion, chopped
- 1 cup vegetable stock
- ½ small-sized cucumber, sliced
- ½ small-sized carrot, sliced
- ¼ tsp salt
- 3 tbsp olive oil
- ½ cup fresh parsley, chopped

Instructions:

1. First, pour the couscous into a large bowl. Boil the vegetable broth and slightly add in the couscous while stirring constantly. Leave it for about 10 minutes until couscous absorbs the liquid. Cover with a lid and set aside. Stir from time to time to speed up the soaking process and break the lumps with a spoon.

2. Meanwhile, preheat the olive oil in a frying pan, and add the tomato sauce. Add chopped onion and stir until translucent. Set aside and let it cool for a few minutes.

3. Add the oily tomato sauce to the couscous and stir well. Now add lemon juice, chopped parsley, and salt to the mixture and give it a final stir.

4. Serve with sliced cucumber, carrot, and parsley.

Nutritional Value Per Serving:

Net carbs 32.8 g

Fiber 3.2 g

Fats 11 g

Sugar 6 g

Calories 249

Lean Spring Stew

Prep time: 20 minutes

Cook time: 1 hour 15 minutes

Serves: 4

Difficulty: Expert

Ingredients:

- 1 lb. diced fire roasted tomatoes
- 4 boneless, skinless chicken thighs
- 1 tbsp dried basil
- 8 oz chicken stock
- Salt & pepper to taste
- 4 oz tomato paste
- 3 chopped celery stalks
- 3 chopped carrots
- 2 chili peppers, finely chopped
- 2 tbsp olive oil
- 1 finely chopped onion
- 2 garlic cloves, crushed
- ½ container mushrooms
- Sour cream

Instructions:

1. Heat up the olive oil over medium-high temperature. Add the celery, onions and carrots and stir-fry for 5 to 10 minutes.

2. Transfer to a deep pot and add tomato paste, basil, garlic, mushrooms and seasoning. Keep stirring the vegetables until they are completely covered by tomato sauce. At the same time, cut the chicken into small cubes to make it easier to eat.

3. Put the chicken in a deep pot, pour the chicken stock over it and throw in the tomatoes.

4. Stir the chicken in to ensure the ingredients and vegetables are properly mixed with it. Turn the heat to low and cook for about an hour. The vegetables and chicken should be cooked through before you turn the heat off. Top with sour cream and serve!

Nutritional Value Per Serving:

Net carbs 19 g

Fiber 5.3 g

Fats 11.9 g

Sugar 3 g

Calories 277

Orange Arugula Salad with Smoked Turkey

Prep time: 10-15 minutes

Serves: 4

Difficulty: Intermediate

Ingredients:

- 3 oz arugula, torn
- 4 oz lamb's lettuce, torn
- 4 oz lettuce, torn

- 8 oz smoked turkey breast, chopped into bite-sized pieces
- 2 large oranges, peeled, sliced

For dressing:

- ¼ cup Greek yogurt
- 3 tbsp lemon juice

- 1 tsp apple cider vinegar
- ¼ cup olive oil

Instructions:

1. Combine arugula, lamb's lettuce, and lettuce in a large colander. Wash thoroughly under cold running water and drain well. Tear into small pieces and set aside.

2. Now, combine vegetables in a large bowl. Add turkey breast and toss well. Then add sliced oranges and set aside.

3. Place Greek yogurt in a small bowl. Add lemon juice, apple cider, and olive oil. Whisk together until fully combined.

4. Drizzle over salad and serve.

Nutritional Value Per Serving:

Net carbs 16.4 g

Fiber 3.1 g

Fats 15.1 g

Sugar 4 g

Calories 231

Dinner
Avocado Eggs with Dried Rosemary

Prep time: 10 minutes

Cook time: 20 minutes

Serves: 6

Difficulty: Expert

Ingredients:

- 3 medium ripe avocados, cut in half, and pit removed
- 6 large eggs
- 1 medium tomato, finely chopped
- 3 tbsp olive oil
- 2 tsp dried rosemary
- ¼ tsp salt
- ¼ tsp black pepper, ground

Instructions:

1. Preheat oven to 350 degrees.
2. Cut avocado in half and remove the pit and flesh from the center. Place one boiled egg and chopped tomato in each avocado half and sprinkle with rosemary, salt and pepper.
3. Grease the baking pan with olive oil and place the avocados on top. You will want to use a small baking pan so your avocados can fit tightly. Place in the oven for about 15-20 minutes.
4. Remove from the oven and let it cool for a while before serving.

Nutritional Value Per Serving:

Net carbs 4 g

Fiber 2.4 g

Fats 16.5 g

Sugar 4 g

Calories 185

Sweet Potatoes with Egg Whites

Prep time: 15 minutes

Cook time: 35-40 minutes

Serves: 4

Difficulty: Intermediate

Ingredients:

- 4 medium sweet potatoes, peeled
- 6 large eggs
- 2 medium onions, peeled
- 1 tbsp ground garlic
- 4 tbsp olive oil
- ½ tsp sea salt
- ¼ tsp ground pepper

Instructions:

1. Preheat your oven to 350 degrees.

2. Spread 2 tablespoons of olive oil over a medium sized baking sheet. Place the potatoes on the baking sheet. Bake for about 20 minutes.

3. Remove from the oven and allow it to cool for a while. Lower the oven heat to 200 degrees.

4. Meanwhile, chop the onions into small pieces. Separate egg whites from yolks. Cut the potatoes into thick slices and place them in a bowl.

5. Add chopped onions, 2 tablespoons of olive oil, egg whites, ground garlic, sea salt and pepper. Mix well.

6. Spread this mixture over a baking sheet and bake for another 15-20 minutes.

Nutritional Value Per Serving:

Net carbs 14.2 g

Fiber 2 g

Fats 21.6 g

Sugar 2 g

Calories 285

Grilled Veal Steak with Vegetables

Prep time: 20 minutes

Cook time: 35 minutes

Serves: 4

Difficulty: Beginner

Ingredients:

- 1 lb. veal steak, about 1 inch thick

- 1 medium red pepper

- 1 medium green pepper

- 1 small onion, finely chopped

- 3 tbsp olive oil

- Salt and pepper to taste

Instructions:

1. Wash and pat dry the steak with kitchen paper. Heat up the olive oil over medium temperature in a non-stick grill pan and fry for about 20 minutes (about 10 on each side). Remove from the heat and set aside.

2. Wash and cut vegetables into thin strips. Add some salt and pepper. Add to a grill pan and cook for about 15 minutes, stirring constantly.

3. Serve immediately.

Nutritional Value Per Serving:

Net carbs 5.3 g

Fiber 1.3 g

Fats 18.5 g

Sugar 2 g

Calories 311

Vegetables in Wok

Prep time: 25 minutes

Cook time: 20 minutes

Serves: 4

Difficulty: Intermediate

Ingredients:

- 1 lb. chicken breast, boneless and skinless
- 1 medium red pepper, cut into strips
- 1 medium green pepper, cut into strips
- 7-8 pieces baby corn
- ½ cup canned button mushrooms
- 1 cup cauliflower
- 1 medium carrot, peeled and cut into strips
- 1 tsp tomato sauce, sugar-free
- Salt to taste
- 1 tbsp olive oil

Instructions:

1. Cut the meat into bite size pieces.

2. In a large wok, heat up the olive oil over a high temperature. Add the chicken meat and cook for about 10 minutes, stirring constantly.

3. Remove from the wok. Now cook the vegetables by first adding carrot strips and cauliflower. They take the most time to soften. Then add red and green pepper strips, baby corn, button mushrooms, and tomato sauce.

4. Cook for another 5-7 minutes. You don't want to overcook the vegetables. They have to stay crispy.

5. Add the meat, mix well and serve with rice.

Nutritional Value Per Serving:

Net carbs 57.6 g   Fats 9.7 g   Calories 420

Fiber 9.4 g   Sugar 2 g

Tandoori Chicken

Prep time: 10 minutes

Cook time: 20 minutes

Serves: 6

Difficulty: Expert

Ingredients:

- 1 cup plain yogurt
- ½ cup lemon juice
- 5 crushed garlic cloves
- 2 tbsps. paprika
- 1 tsp. yellow curry powder
- 1 tsp. ground ginger
- 6 skinless chicken breasts
- 6 skewers

Instructions:

1. Set oven to 400 degrees F. In blender, combine red pepper flakes, ginger, curry, paprika, garlic, lemon juice and yogurt, then process into a smooth paste.

2. Add chicken strips evenly onto skewers. Add chicken to a shallow casserole dish then cover with ½ of yogurt mixture.

3. Tightly seal and rest in refrigerator for about 15 minutes.

4. Lightly grease a baking tray, then transfer chicken skewers onto it, and top with remaining yogurt mixture.

5. Set to bake for about 20 minutes until the chicken is fully cooked. Serve and enjoy.

Nutritional Value Per Serving:

Net carbs 6 g

Fiber 3 g

Fats 7.2 g

Sugar 1 g

Calories 177

Turkey Fajitas Bowls

Prep time: 10 minutes

Cook time: 5 minutes

Serves: 4

Difficulty: Intermediate

Ingredients:

- ½ lb. turkey breast
- 2 tbsps. olive oil
- 1 tbsp. lemon juice
- 1 crushed garlic
- ¾ tsp. chopped chili pepper
- ½ tsp. dried oregano

- 1 sliced bell pepper
- 1 medium tomato
- ½ cup shredded cheddar cheese
- 4 tostada bowls
- 4 tbsps. salsa

Instructions:

1. Add oregano, chili pepper, garlic, lemon juice and 1tbsp. olive oil to a medium bowl. Whisk to combine.

2. Add turkey then toss to coat. Allow to marinate for about 30 min.

3. Set a skillet over medium heat with remaining oil. Add bell pepper and allow to cook for 2 minutes, stirring.

4. Add turkey and cook for 3 more minutes. Add tomato, stir and remove from heat.

5. Spoon mixture evenly into tostada bowls.

6. Garnish with cheese and salsa then serve.

Nutritional Value Per Serving:

Net carbs 5 g

Fiber 3 g

Fats 15 g

Sugar 8 g

Calories 240

Skinny Chicken Pesto Bake

Prep time: 5 minutes

Cook time: 20 minutes

Serves: 4

Difficulty: Beginner

Ingredients:

- 160 oz. skinless chicken
- 1 tsps. basil
- 1 sliced tomato
- 6 tbsps. shredded mozzarella cheese
- 2 tsps. grated parmesan cheese

Instructions:

1. Cut chicken into thin strips.
2. Set oven to 400 degrees F. Prepare a baking sheet by lining with parchment paper.
3. Lay chicken strips on prepared baking sheet. Top with pesto and brush evenly over chicken pieces.
4. Set to bake until chicken is fully cooked (about 15 minutes).
5. Garnish with parmesan cheese, mozzarella, and tomatoes.
6. Set to continue baking until cheese melts (about 5 minutes).

Nutritional Value Per Serving:

Net carbs 2.5 g

Fiber 4 g

Fats 8.5 g

Sugar 4 g

Calories 205

Spaghetti Squash Lasagna V

Prep time: 5 minutes

Cook time: 25 minutes

Serves: 6

Difficulty: Expert

Ingredients:

- 2 cup marinara sauce

- 3 cup roasted spaghetti squash

- 1 cup ricotta

- 8 tsps. grated parmesan cheese

- 6 oz. shredded mozzarella cheese

- ¼ tsp. red pepper flakes

Instructions:

1. Set oven to preheat oven to 375 degrees F and spoon half of marinara sauce into baking dish.

2. Top with squash, then layer remaining ingredients.

3. Cover and set to bake until cheese is melted and edges brown (about 20 minutes).

4. Remove cover and return to bake for another 5 minutes. Enjoy!

Nutritional Value Per Serving:

Net carbs 5.5 g

Fiber 5 g

Fats 15.9 g

Sugar 3 g

Calories 255

Crab Mushrooms

Prep time: 5 minutes

Cook time: 5 minutes

Serves: 5

Difficulty: Beginner

Ingredients:

- 5 oz. crab meat
- 5 oz. white mushrooms
- ½ tsp. salt
- ¼ cup fish stock
- 1 tsp. butter
- ¼ tsp. ground coriander
- 1 tsp. dried cilantro
- 1 tsp. butter

Instructions:

1. Chop the crab meat and sprinkle with salt and dried cilantro.
2. Mix the crab meat carefully. Preheat the air fryer to 400 F.
3. Chop the white mushrooms and combine with crab meat.
4. Add fish stock, ground coriander and butter.
5. Transfer the side dish mixture into the air fryer basket tray.
6. Stir gently with the help of a plastic spatula.
7. Cook the side dish for 5 minutes.
8. Rest for 5 minutes. Serve and enjoy!

Nutritional Value Per Serving:

Net carbs 2.6 g

Fiber 1 g

Fats 1.7 g

Sugar 4 g

Calories 56

Loaded Sweet Potatoes

Prep time: 5 minutes

Cook time: 8 minutes

Serves: 4

Difficulty: Intermediate

Ingredients:

- 4 medium sweet potatoes, baked
- ½ cup Greek yogurt
- 1 tsp. taco seasoning
- 1 tsp. olive oil
- 1 diced red pepper

- ½ diced red onion
- 1 1/3 cup canned black beans
- ½ cup Mexican cheese blend
- ¼ cup chopped cilantro
- ½ cup salsa

Instructions:

1. Mix taco seasoning and yogurt well, then set aside.
2. Set a skillet over medium heat with oil to get hot.
3. Add in remaining ingredients, except potatoes, cheese and salsa, and cook for about 8 minutes or until fully heated through.
4. Slightly pierce potatoes down the center and top evenly with all remaining ingredients. Serve.

Nutritional Value Per Serving:

Net carbs 57 g

Fiber 4 g

Fats 8.3 g

Sugar 7 g

Calories 311

Coconut Flour Spinach Casserole

Prep time: 7 minutes

Cook time: 30 minutes

Serves: 6

Difficulty: Intermediate

Ingredients:

- 4 eggs
- ¾ cup unsweetened almond milk
- 3 oz. chopped spinach
- 3 oz. chopped artichoke hearts
- 1 cup grated parmesan
- 3 minced garlic cloves
- 1 tsp. salt
- ½ tsp. pepper
- ¾ cup coconut flour
- 1 tbsp. baking powder

Instructions:

1. Preheat air fryer to 375 degrees F. Grease air fryer pan with cooking spray.
2. Whisk eggs with almond milk, spinach, artichoke hearts and ½ cup of parmesan cheese. Add salt, garlic and pepper.
3. Add the coconut flour and baking powder; whisk until well combined.
4. Spread mixture into air fryer pan and sprinkle remaining cheese over it.
5. Place the baking pan in the air fryer and cook for about 30 minutes.
6. Remove baking pan from air fryer and sprinkle with chopped basil. Slice, then serve and enjoy!

Nutritional Value Per Serving:

Net carbs 2.4 g

Fiber 3 g

Fats 10.3 g

Sugar 7 g

Calories 175.2

Cherry Tomatoes Tilapia Salad

Prep time: 5 minutes

Cook time: 18 minutes

Serves: 3

Difficulty: Beginner

Ingredients:

- 1 cup mixed greens

- 1 cup cherry tomatoes

- 1/3 cup diced red onion

- 1 medium avocado

- 3 tortilla crusted tilapia fillet

Instructions:

1. Spray tilapia fillet with a little bit of cooking spray. Put fillets in air fryer basket. Cook for 18 minutes at about 390° F.

2. Transfer the fillet to a bowl. Toss with tomatoes, greens and red onion. Add the lime dressing and mix again.

3. Serve and enjoy!

Nutritional Value Per Serving:

Net carbs 10.1 g

Fiber 5 g

Fats 8 g

Sugar 3 g

Calories 271

Snacks

Lemon Berry Pudding

Prep time: 10 minutes

Serves: 4

Difficulty: Beginner

Ingredients:

- 1 package sugar-free fat-free lemon instant pudding mix

- 2 cups cold skim milk

- 4 large strawberries, hulled, mashed

Instructions:

1. In a medium bowl, beat pudding mix and milk with an electric hand mixer until thoroughly blended and slightly thickened, about 2 minutes.

2. Add strawberries to pudding mixture and stir until combined.

3. Pour pudding into 4 small bowls and refrigerate until set, about 5 minutes. Serve immediately, or cover and refrigerate for up to 2 days. Enjoy!

Nutritional Value Per

4. Net carbs 6 g

5. Fiber 1 g

6. Fats 12 g

7. Sugar 3 g

8. Calories 78

Avocado Detox Smoothie

Prep time: 10 minutes

Serves: 2

Difficulty: Intermediate

Ingredients:

- ½ avocado, peeled, roughly chopped
- 1 tbsp powdered stevia
- 1 banana, peeled, chopped
- 1 cup baby spinach, torn
- 1 tbsp goji berries
- 1 tbsp flaxseed, ground
- 1 tsp turmeric, ground

Instructions:

1. Peel the avocado and cut in half. Remove the pit and chop one half into small pieces. Wrap the other half in a plastic foil and refrigerate for later.

2. Peel the banana and cut into thin slices. Set aside.

3. Rinse the spinach thoroughly under cold running water using a colander. Chop into small pieces and set aside.

4. Now, combine avocado, banana, spinach, turmeric, flaxseed, and goji berries in a blender. Process until well combined.

5. Transfer to a serving glass and add few ice cubes.

6. Serve immediately.

Nutritional Value Per Serving:

Net carbs 28.6 g

Fiber 7.5 g

Fats 11.8 g

Sugar 4 g

Calories 221

Sweet Pumpkin Pudding

Prep time: 15 minutes

Cook time: 15 minutes

Serves: 4

Difficulty: Intermediate

Ingredients:

- 1 lb. pumpkin, peeled and chopped into bite-sized pieces
- 2 tbsp honey
- ½ cup cornstarch
- 4 cups pumpkin juice, unsweetened
- 1 tsp cinnamon, ground
- 3 cloves, freshly ground

Instructions:

1. Peel and prepare the pumpkin. Scrape out seeds and chop into bite-sized pieces. Set aside.
2. In a small bowl, combine pumpkin juice, honey, orange juice, cinnamon, and cornstarch.
3. Place the pumpkin chops in a large pot and pour the pumpkin juice mixture. Stir well and then finally add cloves. Stir until well incorporated and heat up until almost boiling. Reduce the heat to low and cook for about 15 minutes, or until the mixture thickens.
4. Remove from the heat and transfer to the bowls immediately. Set aside to cool completely and then refrigerate for 15 minutes before serving, or simply chill overnight.

Nutritional Value Per Serving:

Net carbs 56 g

Fiber 4.6 g

Fats 0.9 g

Sugar 6 g

Calories 232

Beet Spinach Salad

Prep time: 20 minutes

Cook time: 40 minutes

Serves: 3

Difficulty: Expert

Ingredients:

- 2 medium-sized beet, trimmed, sliced

- 1 cup fresh spinach, chopped

- 2 spring onions, finely chopped

- 1 small green apple, cored, chopped

- 3 tbsp olive oil

- 2 tbsp fresh lime juice

- 1 tbsp honey, raw

- 1 tsp apple cider vinegar

- 1 tsp salt

Instructions:

1. Wash the beets and trim off the green parts. Set aside.

2. Wash the spinach thoroughly and drain. Cut into small pieces and set aside.

3. Wash the apple and cut lengthwise in half. Remove the core and cut into bite-sized pieces and set aside.

4. Wash the onions and cut into small pieces. Set aside.

5. In a small bowl, combine olive oil, lime juice, honey, vinegar, and salt. Stir until well incorporated and set aside to allow flavors to meld.

6. Place the beets in a deep pot. Pour enough water to cover and cook for about 40 minutes, or until tender. Remove the skin and slice. Set aside.

7. In a large salad bowl, combine beets, spinach, spring onions, and apple. Stir well until combined and drizzle with previously prepared dressing. Give it a good final stir and serve immediately.

Nutritional Value Per Serving:

Net carbs 23.8 g

Fiber 3.6 g

Fats 14.3 g

Sugar 5 g

Calories 215

Grilled Avocado in Curry Sauce

Prep time: 15 minutes

Cook time: 30 minutes

Serves: 2

Difficulty: Intermediate

Ingredients:

- 1 large avocado, chopped
- ¼ cup water
- 1 tbsp curry, ground
- 2 tbsp olive oil

- 1 tsp soy sauce
- 1 tsp fresh parsley, finely chopped
- ¼ tsp red pepper flakes
- ¼ tsp sea salt

Instructions:

1. Peel the avocado and cut lengthwise in half. Remove the pit and cut the remaining avocado into small chunks. Set aside.

2. Heat up the olive oil in a large saucepan over a medium-high temperature.

3. In a small bowl, combine ground curry, soy sauce, parsley, red pepper and sea salt. Add water and cook for about 5 minutes, stirring occasionally.

4. Add chopped avocado, stir well and cook for 3 more minutes, or until all the liquid evaporates. Turn off the heat and cover. Let it stand for about 15-20 minutes before serving.

Nutritional Value Per Serving:

Net carbs 10.8 g

Fiber 7.9 g

Fats 34.1 g

Sugar 4 g

Calories 338

Broccoli Cauliflower Puree

Prep time: 15 minutes

Cook time: 20 minutes

Serves: 2

Difficulty: Intermediate

Ingredients:

- 2 cups fresh broccoli chopped
- 2 cups fresh cauliflower, chopped
- ½ cup skim milk
- ½ tsp salt
- ½ tsp Italian seasoning
- ¼ tsp cumin, ground
- 1 tbsp fresh parsley, finely chopped
- 1 tbsp olive oil
- 1 tsp dry mint, ground

Instructions:

1. Wash and roughly chop the cauliflower. Place it in a deep pot and add a pinch of salt. Cook for about 15-20 minutes. When done, drain and transfer it to a food processor. Set aside.

2. Wash the broccoli and chop into bite-sized pieces. Add it to the food processor along with milk, salt, Italian seasoning, cumin, parsley, and mint. Gradually add olive oil and blend until nicely pureed.

3. Serve with some fresh carrots and celery.

Nutritional Value Per Serving:

Net carbs 12.7 g

Fiber 4.6 g

Fats 7.5 g

Sugar 2 g

Calories 138

Ginger Peach Smoothie

Prep time: 5 minutes

Serves: 4

Difficulty: Beginner

Ingredients:

- 1 cup coconut milk
- 1 large peach, chopped
- 1 tbsp coconut oil
- 1 tbsp chia seeds
- 1 tsp fresh ginger, peeled

Instructions:

1. Wash the peach and cut into half. Remove the pit and chop into bite-sized pieces. Set aside.

2. Cut small ginger knob. Peel it and chop into small pieces. Set aside.

3. Now, combine peach, ginger, coconut milk, and coconut oil in a blender. Process until well combined. Transfer to a serving glass and stir in the chia seeds.

4. Enjoy!

Nutritional Value Per Serving:

Net carbs 8.9 g

Fiber 3.5 g

Fats 19 g

Sugar 6 g

Calories 201

Red Orange Salad

Prep time: 15 minutes

Cook time: 20 minutes

Serves: 3

Difficulty: Intermediate

Ingredients:

- Fresh lettuce leaves, rinsed
- 1 small cucumber sliced
- ½ red bell pepper, sliced
- 1 cup frozen seafood mix
- 1 onion, peeled, finely chopped
- 3 garlic cloves, crushed
- ¼ cup fresh orange juice
- 5 tbsp extra virgin olive oil
- Salt to taste

Instructions:

1. Heat up 3 tbsp of extra virgin olive oil over medium-high temperature. Add chopped onion and crushed garlic. Stir fry for about 5 minutes.

2. Reduce the heat to minimum and add 1 cup of frozen seafood mix. Cover and cook for about 15 minutes, until soft. Remove from the heat and allow it to cool for a while.

3. Meanwhile, combine the vegetables in a bowl. Add the remaining 2 tbsp of olive oil, fresh orange juice and a little salt. Toss well to combine.

4. Top with seafood mix and serve immediately.

Nutritional Value Per Serving:

Net carbs 13.1 g

Fiber 1.8 g

Fats 14.6 g

Sugar 4 g

Calories 206

Fresh Mango Smoothie

Prep time: 10 minutes

Serves: 3

Difficulty: Beginner

Ingredients:

- 1 medium mango, roughly chopped

- 1 cup coconut milk

- 1 tbsp walnuts, chopped

- 1 tsp vanilla extract, sugar-free

- A handful of ice cubes

Instructions:

1. Peel the mango and cut into small chunks. Set aside.

2. Now, combine mango, coconut milk, walnuts, and vanilla extract in a blender and process until well combined and creamy. Transfer to a serving glass and stir in the vanilla extract. Add a few ice cubes and serve immediately.

Nutritional Value Per Serving:

Net carbs 21.7 g

Fiber 3.7 g

Fats 21 g

Sugar 4 g

Calories 271

Poultry

Chicken Thighs

Prep time: 20 minutes

Cook time: 40 minutes

Serves: 6

Difficulty: Expert

Ingredients:

- 2 lbs. chicken thighs
- 2 medium onions, chopped
- 2 small chili peppers
- 1 cup chicken broth
- ¼ cup freshly squeezed orange juice, unsweetened
- 1 tsp orange extract, sugar-free
- 2 tbsp olive oil
- 1 tsp barbecue seasoning mix
- 1 small red onion, chopped

Instructions:

1. Heat up the olive oil in a large saucepan. Add chopped onions and fry for several minutes, over a medium temperature – until golden color.

2. Combine chili peppers, orange juice and orange extract. Mix well in a food processor for 20-30 seconds. Add this mixture into a saucepan and stir well. Reduce heat to simmer.

3. Coat the chicken with barbecue seasoning mix and put into a saucepan. Add chicken broth and bring it to boil. Cook over a medium temperature until the water evaporates. Remove from the heat.

4. Preheat the oven to 350 degrees. Place the chicken into a large baking dish. Bake for about 15 minutes to get a nice crispy, golden brown color.

Nutritional Value Per Serving:

Net carbs 5.2 g

Fiber 0.9 g

Fats 16.2 g

Sugar 3 g

Calories 357

Chicken Cordon Bleu

Prep time: 16 minutes

Cook time: 30 minutes

Serves: 5

Difficulty: Intermediate

Ingredients:

- 6 chicken breasts, skinless, boneless, thinly sliced
- 6 slices lean deli ham
- 6 slices reduced-fat Swiss cheese, halved

- 2 large eggs
- 1 tablespoon water
- ½ cup whole wheat bread crumbs
- 2 tablespoons Parmigiano-Reggiano cheese

Instructions:

1. Pre-heat your oven to 450 degrees F.
2. Spray a baking sheet with cooking spray, pound chicken breasts to ¼ inch thickness.
3. Layer 1 slice ham and 1 slice (2 halves) cheese on each chicken breast.
4. Roll chicken and transfer them to the baking sheet (seam side down).
5. Take a small bowl and add whisk in eggs, take another bowl and mix in bread crumbs and cheese.
6. Use a pastry brush and lightly brush each chicken roll with egg wash. Sprinkle bread crumbs all over.
7. Bake for 30 minutes until the top is lightly browned.
8. Enjoy!

Nutritional Value Per Serving:

Net carbs 3 g

Fiber 1 g

Fats 7 g

Sugar 4 g

Calories 174

Creamy Chicken Soup And Cauliflower

Prep time: 15 minutes

Cook time: 40 minutes

Serves: 4

Difficulty: Expert

Ingredients:

- 1 teaspoon garlic, minced
- 1 teaspoon extra virgin olive oil
- ½ yellow onion, diced
- 1 carrot, diced
- 1 celery stalk, diced
- 1 and ½ pounds cooked chicken breast, diced
- 2 cups low sodium chicken broth
- 2 cups of water
- 1 teaspoon fresh ground black pepper
- 1 teaspoon dried thyme
- 2 and ½ cups fresh cauliflower florets
- 1 cup fresh spinach, chopped
- 2 cups nonfat milk

Instructions:

1. Place large soup over medium-high heat and add garlic in olive oil, Sauté for 1 minute.

2. Add onion, carrot, celery, Sauté for 3-5 minutes.

3. Add chicken breast, broth, water, pepper, thyme, cauliflower and simmer over low-medium heat, cover and cook for 30 minutes.

4. Add fresh spinach and stir for 5 minutes.

5. Stir in milk and serve, enjoy!

Nutritional Value Per Serving:

Net carbs 5 g

Fiber 1 g

Fats 3 g

Sugar 2 g

Calories 164

Grilled Chicken Wings

Prep time: 15 minutes

Cook time: 20 minutes

Serves: 6

Difficulty: Beginner

Ingredients:

- 1 and ½ pounds frozen chicken wings
- Fresh ground black pepper
- 1 teaspoon garlic powder
- 1 cup buffalo

Instructions:

1. Pre-heat your grill to 350 degrees F.
2. Season wings with pepper and garlic powder, grill wings for 15 minutes per side.
3. Once they are browned and crispy, toss grilled wings in Buffalo wings sauce and olive oil.
4. Enjoy!

Nutritional Value Per Serving:

Net carbs 1 g

Fiber 3 g

Fats 6 g

Sugar 2 g

Calories 82

Buffalo Chicken Wrap

Prep time: 10 minutes

Serves: 4

Difficulty: Beginner

Ingredients:

- 3 cups rotisserie chicken breast
- 2 cups romaine lettuce, chopped
- 1 tomato, diced
- ½ red onion, finely sliced
- ¼ cup buffalo wing sauce
- ¼ cup creamy peppercorn ranch dressing
- Chopped raw celery as for garnish
- 5 small whole grain low carb wraps

Instructions:

1. Take a large mixing bowl and add chicken, lettuce, tomato, onion, wing sauce, dressing, and celery.
2. Add 1 cup of mixture onto each wrap and foil wrap over the salad.
3. Use a toothpick to secure the wrap, enjoy!

Nutritional Value Per Serving:

Net carbs 14 g

Fiber 3 g

Fats 7 g

Sugar 1 g

Calories 200

Chicken Cauliflower Bowls

Prep time: 20 minutes

Cook time: 12 minutes

Serves: 4

Difficulty: Expert

Ingredients:

- 1 large head cauliflower, cored
- 1/2 cup chicken stock
- 1 teaspoon butter
- 1/4 cup chopped onion
- 1/4 cup chopped bell pepper
- 1 cup chopped cooked chicken breast
- 1 teaspoon garlic powder
- Salt and freshly ground black pepper, to taste
- 1/4 cup shredded white cheddar cheese

Instructions:

1. Pour water into a large saucepan to a depth of about 2 inches. Set steamer basket in saucepan and place cauliflower in basket. Cover pan and steam over medium heat until cauliflower is soft, 10 to 12 minutes.

2. Meanwhile, heat butter in a medium nonstick skillet and sauté onion and bell pepper until softened, 4 to 5 minutes, stirring frequently. Remove skillet from heat, add cooked chicken and garlic powder, season to taste with salt and pepper and stir to combine.

3. Carefully remove cauliflower from steamer basket and place in a large bowl. Crumble and lightly mash cauliflower with a fork and season to taste with salt and pepper. Add chicken stock to cauliflower and puree with an immersion blender until smooth, adding more stock if needed.

4. Scoop cauliflower into 4 bowls, top with the chicken mixture and sprinkle with the grated cheese to serve. Enjoy!

Nutritional Value Per Serving:

Net carbs 13 g

Fiber 6 g

Fats 5 g

Sugar 4 g

Calories 149

Chicken Caprese

Prep time: 15 minutes

Cook time: 15 minutes

Serves: 4

Difficulty: Expert

Ingredients:

- 1 pound boneless skinless chicken breasts
- 2 tablespoons olive oil, divided
- 1 teaspoon garlic powder
- 1 teaspoon onion powder
- 1 teaspoon Italian herb seasoning
- Salt and freshly ground black pepper
- 1/2 cup grated mozzarella cheese
- 1 cup halved cherry tomatoes
- 2 tablespoons balsamic vinegar
- 2 tablespoons sliced fresh basil leaves

Instructions:

1. Cut chicken breasts lengthwise into 1" thick slices and brush all over with about 1 tablespoon olive oil. Mix garlic powder, onion powder and herb seasoning, sprinkle over chicken and season to taste with salt and pepper.

2. Heat remaining 1 tablespoon olive oil in a large nonstick skillet over medium heat and cook chicken until lightly golden brown and no longer pink inside, 8 to 10 minutes,

turning as necessary. Sprinkle mozzarella cheese over chicken and cook until cheese is melted, about 1 minute more.

3. Transfer chicken to a serving plate and arrange tomatoes over chicken. Drizzle balsamic vinegar over chicken, sprinkle with basil and serve immediately. Enjoy!

Nutritional Value Per Serving:

Net carbs 3 g

Fiber 1 g

Fats 9 g

Sugar 4 g

Calories 170

Pulled Chicken

Prep time: 15 minutes

Cook time: 8 to 10 hours

Serves: 3

Difficulty: Intermediate

Ingredients:

- 1 small onion, cut into strips

- 1 small bell pepper, strips

- 1 garlic clove, minced

- 1 tablespoon taco seasoning or barbecue spice rub

- 2 boneless skinless chicken breasts

Instructions:

1. Arrange onion and bell pepper strips in the bottom of a 3- to 4-quart slow cooker and sprinkle with garlic.

2. Rub chicken breasts all over with taco seasoning and place in slow cooker.

3. Cover slow cooker and cook chicken on low until cooked through and tender, 8 to 10 hours.

4. Remove chicken from slow cooker and shred with two forks. Add juices from slow cooker to chicken and sprinkle with additional taco seasoning if desired. Serve immediately and enjoy!

Nutritional Value Per Serving:

Net carbs 7 g

Fiber 1 g

Fats 3 g

Sugar 2 g

Calories 142

Lemon Chicken

Prep time: 20 minutes

Cook time: 20 minutes

Serves: 3

Difficulty: Expert

Ingredients:

- 2 teaspoons olive oil
- 2 boneless skinless chicken breasts
- 2 garlic cloves, minced
- 1 cup chicken stock
- 2 lemons, zested, juiced
- 1 teaspoon lemon pepper seasoning
- 1/2 teaspoon dried basil
- 1/2 teaspoon dried oregano
- Salt and freshly ground black pepper
- 1 tablespoon cornstarch
- 2 tablespoons cold water

Instructions:

1. Heat olive oil in a large nonstick skillet over medium heat and sauté chicken just until cooked through, 7 to 8 minutes, stirring frequently. Add garlic and sauté about 1 minute more, stirring constantly.

2. Add chicken stock, lemon juice, lemon pepper, basil and oregano to chicken mixture and season to taste with salt and pepper. Reduce heat and simmer until chicken is cooked through and liquid is slightly reduced, 7 to 8 minutes, stirring occasionally.

3. Whisk cornstarch into cold water, add to skillet and stir gently until combined. Simmer until sauce is thickened, about 2 minutes, stirring constantly.

4. Transfer lemon chicken to a large bowl, sprinkle with lemon zest and serve immediately. Enjoy!

Nutritional Value Per Serving:

Net carbs 8 g   Fats 5 g   Calories 134

Fiber 1 g   Sugar 2 g

Turkey Soup

Prep time: 20 minutes

Cook time: 30 minutes

Serves: 6

Difficulty: Expert

Ingredients:

- 1 tablespoon butter
- 1 pound boneless skinless turkey thighs
- 6 cups chicken stock
- 1/2 teaspoon kosher salt, plus more to taste
- 1/4 teaspoon freshly ground black pepper
- 2 celery stalks, diced
- 2 carrots, peeled, diced
- 1 small onion, diced
- 1 1/2 teaspoons dried Italian herb seasoning
- 2 dried bay leaves

Instructions:

1. Melt butter in a stock pot or large saucepan over medium heat and sauté turkey thighs until browned on all sides, about 5 minutes.

2. Add chicken stock, salt and pepper to pot and heat to a boil. Reduce heat, cover pot and simmer for about 10 minutes.

3. Add celery, carrots, onion, herb seasoning and bay leaves to pot, season to taste with salt and pepper and stir to combine. Cover pot and simmer until vegetables are tender, about 15 minutes more.

4. Remove bay leaves from soup and discard. Remove turkey thighs from soup, cut into bite-size pieces and stir back into soup. Serve soup immediately and enjoy!

Nutritional Value Per Serving:

Net carbs 4 g   Fats 7 g   Calories 139

Fiber 1 g   Sugar 4 g

Chicken Curry Wraps

Prep time: 10 minutes

Serves: 2

Difficulty: Intermediate

Ingredients:

- 1 cup cooked diced chicken
- 1/2 cup plain unsweetened yogurt
- 1 tablespoon skim milk, plus more if needed
- 1 celery stalk, diced
- 1/2 teaspoon curry powder
- 1/4 teaspoon onion powder
- Salt and freshly ground black pepper
- 2 large green lettuce leaves
- 1 tablespoon slivered almonds, toasted

Instructions:

1. Mix chicken, yogurt, milk, celery, curry powder and onion powder and season to taste with salt and pepper.

2. Spread chicken mixture on lettuce leaves and sprinkle with almonds.

3. Roll up lettuce leaves burrito-style over chicken mixture. Serve immediately and enjoy!

Nutritional Value Per Serving:

Net carbs 3 g

Fiber 1 g

Fats 5 g

Sugar 3 g

Calories 148

Pork

Roasted Pork Tenderloin Puree

Prep time: 20 minutes

Cook time: 25 minutes

Serves: 10

Difficulty: Expert

Ingredients:

- 1 pork tenderloin
- 1 teaspoon kosher salt
- 1/2 teaspoon freshly ground black pepper
- 1 teaspoon Italian herb seasoning
- 1 teaspoon ground coriander
- 1/2 teaspoon garlic powder
- 1/2 teaspoon onion powder
- 1 teaspoon vegetable oil
- 3/4 cup vegetable or chicken stock

Instructions:

1. Place a medium cast iron or oven-safe skillet in the oven. Preheat oven to 450°F.

2. Mix salt, pepper, Italian herb seasoning, coriander, garlic powder and onion powder and set aside.

3. Trim fat and silver skin from pork tenderloin as necessary and pat tenderloin dry with paper towels. Pierce tenderloin all over with a fork and evenly rub with spice mixture.

4. Using oven mitts, carefully remove hot skillet from the oven. Drizzle oil into skillet and swirl gently to coat. Place tenderloin in skillet, return to oven and roast for 10 minutes.

Flip tenderloin, reduce oven temperature to 400°F and roast until the internal temperature of the tenderloin reaches 145°F, 10 to 15 minutes more.

5. Transfer tenderloin to a serving plate, cover loosely with aluminum foil and let rest for about 10 minutes. Cut tenderloin into 1" thick slices, cover tightly and refrigerate until chilled through, about 2 hours.

6. Cut chilled tenderloin slices into 1" cubes. Place about 1 cup tenderloin cubes in a food processor and pulse until fine and powdery (the texture should resemble sand). Add about 1/4 cup stock and process until smooth. Repeat with remaining tenderloin cubes.

7. Season pureed tenderloin to taste with salt and pepper and stir until thoroughly combined.

8. Pureed tenderloin can be served immediately. Or, divide pureed tenderloin into 1/2-cup portions in zip-top plastic bags or tightly covered containers, and store in the refrigerator for up to 4 days or in the freezer for up to 2 weeks. Reheat cold tenderloin puree in the microwave before serving. Enjoy!

Nutritional Value Per Serving:

Net carbs 1 g

Fiber 2 g

Fats 6 g

Sugar 4 g

Calories 142

Chipotle Shredded Pork

Prep time: 10 minutes

Cook time: 6 hours 10 minutes

Serves: 8

Difficulty: Intermediate

Ingredients:

- 1 can chipotle pepper in adobo sauce
- 1 ½ tablespoon apple cider vinegar
- 1 tablespoon ground cumin
- 1 tablespoon dried oregano
- Juice of 1 lime
- 2 pounds pork shoulder, trimmed

Instructions:

1. Take your blender and puree chipotle pepper, adobo sauce, apple cider vinegar, cumin, oregano, and lime juice.

2. Transfer pork shoulder in the slow cooker and pour the sauce all over.

3. Cover Slow Cooker and cook for 6 hours on low.

4. Shred the pork using forks and enjoy!

Nutritional Value Per Serving:

Net carbs 5 g

Fiber 1 g

Fats 11 g

Sugar 3 g

Calories 260

Brown Sugar-Mustard Pork Chops

Prep time: 15 minutes

Cook time: 30 minutes

Serves: 6

Difficulty: Beginner

Ingredients:

- 6 Boneless pork loin chops
- ¼ cup, Yellow mustard
- ½ cup, Brown sugar

Instructions:

1. In a medium bowl, mix brown sugar and mustard.
2. Wash and clean the pork.
3. Take glass baking tray and spray some non-stick cooking oil.
4. Place the cleaned pork in the tray.
5. Transfer the mix over the pork chops.
6. Set the temperature of the baking oven at 350°F and bake the pork for 30 minutes.
7. Once ready, serve hot.

Nutritional Value Per Serving:

Net carbs 12.6 g

Fiber 0.5 g

Fats 6.5 g

Sugar 7 g

Calories 298

Balsamic-Glazed Pork Tenderloin

Prep time: 10 minutes

Cook time: 25 minutes

Serves: 6

Difficulty: Intermediate

Ingredients:

- 1½ pound, Pork tenderloin
- 3 tablespoons, Brown sugar
- ¼ teaspoon, Salt
- 1/8 teaspoon, Black pepper
- ¼ cup, Balsamic vinegar
- 2 tablespoons, Cooking oil

Instructions:

1. Wash and clean pork.
2. Pat dry and season the pork with pepper and salt.
3. Set the oven to 425°F.
4. In a skillet pour cooking oil and roast the pork to brown in medium-low heat.
5. Once all the pork turns brown from all side, remove it.
6. Now add balsamic vinegar and add brown sugar.
7. Stir continuously and let all the brown bits remove from the skillet and becomes a glaze.
8. Now put back the pork into the skillet and allow the glaze to coat evenly on the pork piece.
9. Transfer the entire pork coated with brown sugar and balsamic vinegar into a roasting pan and bake it for about 25 minutes.
10. Spread the glaze over the pork frequently.

96

11. Serve hot.

Nutritional Value Per Serving:

Net carbs 4.5 g

Fiber 1 g

Fats 2 g

Sugar 3 g

Calories 222

Pork Chops with Honey & Garlic

Prep time: 5 minutes

Cook time: 20 minutes

Serves: 6

Difficulty: Beginner

Ingredients:

- 24 ounces, Pork loin chops, fat removed, cut into 6 pieces.
- 1/8 +¼ cup, Honey
- 3 tablespoons, Soy sauce
- 6 cloves, Garlic, finely chopped

Instructions:

1. Combine soy sauce, ¼ cup honey, and garlic in a medium bowl.
2. Marinate the chops in the mixture.
3. Bring grill to medium-high temperature and place chops over it.
4. Cover and cook for 20 minutes.
5. Sprinkle the remaining honey over the chops while grilling.

Nutritional Value Per Serving:

Net carbs 24.9

Fiber 0.2 g

Fats 5.9 g

Sugar 2 g

Calories 369

Vegetables

Avocado Pineapple Salad

Prep time: 20 minutes

Serves: 3

Difficulty: Intermediate

Ingredients:

- 1 cup avocado chunks
- 1 cup pineapple chunks
- 1 cup watermelon
- 1 cup sour cream
- 1 cup spinach, finely chopped
- 1 tbsp honey
- 1 tsp vanilla extract
- 1 tbsp flaxseeds

Instructions:

1. In a medium bowl, combine sour cream, honey, vanilla extract, and flaxseeds. Stir well to combine and set aside.

2. Wash and prepare the vegetables.

3. Peel the avocado and pineapple and cut in half. Remove the pit from the avocado and cut into small chunks along with pineapple. Place in a large salad bowl and set aside.

4. Cut one large watermelon wedge and peel it. Cut into bite-sized pieces and discard the seeds. Add it to the bowl with other fruits and set aside.

5. Wash the spinach thoroughly under cold running water and roughly chop it. Add it to the bowl with other fruits.

6. Now, pour the sour cream mixture over the fruits and veggies and toss well to coat all the ingredients.

7. Refrigerate for 15 minutes before serving.

Nutritional Value Per Serving:

Net carbs 26.3 g

Fiber 5.8 g

Fats 25.9 g

Sugar 2 g

Calories 343

Fresh Tomato and Celery Soup

Prep time: 10 minutes

Cook time: 30 minutes

Serves: 4

Difficulty: Expert

Ingredients:

- 1 lb. tomatoes, peeled, roughly chopped

- 4 oz celery root, finely chopped

- ¼ cup fresh celery leaves, finely chopped

- 1 tbsp fresh basil, finely chopped

- Salt and pepper

- 5 tbsp extra virgin olive oil

Instructions:

1. Preheat the oil in a large non-stick frying pan over a medium-high temperature. Add finely chopped celery root, celery leaves, and fresh basil. Season with salt and pepper and stir-fry for about 10 minutes, until nicely browned.

2. Add chopped tomatoes and about ¼ cup of water. Reduce the heat to minimum and cook for 15 minutes, stirring constantly, until softened. Now add about 4 cups of water (or vegetable broth) and bring it to a boil. Give it a good stir and remove from the heat.

3. Top with fresh parsley and serve.

Nutritional Value Per Serving:

Net carbs 6.9 g

Fiber 1.9 g

Fats 10.8 g

Sugar 2 g

Calories 122

Saucy Garlic Broccoli

Prep time: 15 minutes

Cook time: 15 minutes

Serves: 4

Difficulty: Intermediate

Ingredients:

- 2 stalks broccoli

- Salt and freshly ground black pepper

- 1 tablespoon olive oil

- 2 garlic cloves, minced

- 1 tablespoon ginger, minced

- 2 cups chicken stock

- 2 tablespoons soy sauce

- 1/2 teaspoon red pepper flakes

- 2 tablespoons cornstarch

- 1/4 cup chopped salted cashews

Instructions:

1. Pour water into a large saucepan to a depth of about 2 inches. Set steamer basket in saucepan, place broccoli in basket and season to taste with salt and pepper. Cover pan and steam over medium heat until broccoli is soft, 8 to 10 minutes.

2. Transfer broccoli to a serving dish, cover to keep warm and set aside. Empty cooking water from pan.

3. For the sauce, in the same pan, heat oil over medium heat and sauté garlic and ginger for about 1 minute. Add chicken broth, soy sauce and red pepper flakes to pan, season to taste with salt and pepper and heat to a simmer, stirring occasionally, about 10 minutes.

4. Dissolve cornstarch in about 1/4 cup cold water, whisk into sauce and cook until sauce is thickened, stirring constantly, about 2 minutes.

5. Pour sauce over broccoli and stir gently to coat. Sprinkle cashews over broccoli and serve immediately. Enjoy!

Nutritional Value Per Serving:

Net carbs 32 g

Fiber 3 g

Fats 12 g

Sugar 1 g

Calories 232

Lemon Avocado Soup

Prep time: 15 minutes

Serves: 4

Difficulty: Beginner

Ingredients:

- 2 avocados, pitted, peeled, diced
- 1 small onion, diced
- 2 garlic cloves, minced
- 2 tablespoons chopped chipotles in adobo sauce
- 1 1/2 cups plain unsweetened Greek yogurt
- 3/4 cup skim milk
- 1 lemon, zested, juiced
- 1 teaspoon ground cumin
- 1 teaspoon kosher salt
- Chili powder, for garnish

Instructions:

1. Pulse avocados, onion, garlic and chipotles in a food processor until thoroughly combined. Add yogurt, milk, lemon juice, cumin and salt and process until smooth. Add milk as necessary to achieve desired consistency.

2. Refrigerate soup until chilled through, about 1 hour.

3. Ladle soup into 4 bowls and sprinkle with lemon zest and chili powder to serve. Enjoy!

Nutritional Value Per Serving:

Net carbs 20 g

Fiber 7 g

Fats 19 g

Sugar 1 g

Calories 262

Mashed Cauliflower

Prep time: 20 minutes

Cook time: 12 minutes

Serves: 4

Difficulty: Intermediate

Ingredients:

- 1 large head cauliflower, cored

- 1/2 cup skim milk

- 1/4 teaspoon garlic powder

- 1/4 teaspoon onion powder

- Salt and freshly ground black pepper

Instructions:

1. Pour water into a large saucepan to a depth of about 2 inches. Set steamer basket in saucepan and place cauliflower in basket. Cover pan and steam over medium heat until cauliflower is soft, 10 to 12 minutes.

2. Carefully remove cauliflower from steamer basket and place in a large bowl. Crumble and lightly mash cauliflower with a fork.

3. Add milk, garlic powder and onion powder to cauliflower and puree with an immersion blender until smooth or to desired consistency, adding more milk if needed.

4. Season cauliflower to taste with salt and pepper and serve . Enjoy!

Nutritional Value Per Serving:

Net carbs 13 g

Fiber 5 g

Fats 1 g

Sugar 1 g

Calories 64

Mini Vegetable Frittatas

Prep time: 15 minutes

Cook time: 15 minutes

Serves: 9

Difficulty: Intermediate

Ingredients:

- 5 Eggs
- 2 ounces Goat cheese, shredded
- 2 tablespoons Low-fat milk
- 1 cup Tomato, chopped
- 2 cups Chopped broccoli, fresh

Ingredients from the kitchen store:

- ¼ teaspoon Pepper crushed
- ¼ teaspoon Salt
- Cooking spray

Instructions:

1. Blend milk and eggs in a mixer bowl.
2. Add crumbled goat cheese and all the chopped vegetables in it and combine.
3. Season it with pepper and salt.
4. Spoon this mixture into muffin cups sprayed with cooking oil.
5. Bake it at 350°F for about 12-15 minutes until it becomes golden color on the top.
6. Serve hot.

Nutritional Value Per Serving:

Net carbs 3.9 g

Fiber 1.4 g

Fats 4.03 g

Sugar 1 g

Calories 71.3

Fish and seafood

Easy Baked Salmon

Prep time: 5 minutes

Cook time: 15 minutes

Serves: 4

Difficulty: Intermediate

Ingredients:

- 4 salmon fillets
- 1 lemon zest
- 1 tsp sea salt
- 3 oz olive oil

- 1 garlic clove, minced
- 1 tsp fresh dill, chopped
- 1 tbsp fresh parsley, chopped
- 1/8 tsp white pepper

Instructions:

1. Preheat the oven at 200 C.
2. Place all ingredients except salmon fillet in microwave safe bowl and microwave for 45 seconds.
3. Stir well until combine.
4. Place salmon fillets on parchment lined baking dish.
5. Spread evenly olive oil and herb mixture over the each salmon fillet.
6. Place in preheated oven and bake for 15 minutes.
7. Serve and enjoy.

Nutritional Value Per Serving:

Net carbs 0.5 g

Fiber 3.1 g

Fats 30.9 g

Sugar 1 g

Calories 408

Wild Salmon Salad

Prep time: 10 minutes

Serves: 2

Difficulty: Intermediate

Ingredients:

- 2 medium-sized cucumbers, sliced
- A handful of iceberg lettuce, torn
- ¼ cup sweet corn
- 1 large tomato, roughly chopped
- 8 oz smoked wild salmon, sliced
- 4 tbsp freshly squeezed orange juice

Dressing:

- 1 ¼ cup liquid yogurt, 2% fat
- 1 tbsp fresh mint, finely chopped
- 2 garlic cloves, crushed
- 1 tbsp sesame seeds

Instructions:

1. Combine vegetables in a large bowl. Drizzle with orange juice and top with salmon slices. Set aside.

2. In another bowl, whisk together yogurt, mint, crushed garlic, and sesame seeds.

3. Drizzle over salad and toss to combine. Serve cold.

Nutritional Value Per Serving:

Net carbs 32.8 g

Fiber 3.2 g

Fats 11 g

Sugar 2 g

Calories 249

Herbed Salmon

Prep time: 10 minutes

Cook time: 15 minutes

Serves: 2

Difficulty: Expert

Ingredients:

- 2 salmon fillets

- 1/2 teaspoon onion powder

- 1/2 teaspoon garlic powder

- Salt and freshly ground black pepper

- 1 tablespoon olive oil

- 1 can diced tomatoes

- 1 teaspoon Italian herb seasoning

- 2 tablespoons finely grated Parmesan cheese

Instructions:

1. Preheat a medium nonstick skillet over medium heat. Brush salmon fillets with olive oil, sprinkle with onion and garlic powder and season to taste with salt and pepper. Sear fillets until browned on both sides, turning as necessary, 3 to 4 minutes

2. Pour undrained tomatoes over salmon fillets, sprinkle with herb seasoning and season to taste with salt and pepper. Heat to a boil, then reduce heat, cover and simmer until salmon is cooked through, 6 to 8 minutes.

3. Transfer salmon with sauce onto plates and sprinkle with Parmesan cheese to serve. Enjoy!

Nutritional Value Per Serving:

Net carbs 7 g

Fiber 2 g

Fats 10 g

Sugar 1 g

Calories 227

Slowly Roasted Pesto Salmon

Prep time: 5 minutes

Cook time: 20 minutes

Serves: 4

Difficulty: Beginner

Ingredients:

- 4 salmon fillets
- 1 teaspoon extra-virgin olive oil
- 4 tablespoons basil pesto

Instructions:

1. Pre-heat your oven to 275 degrees F.
2. Line a rimmed baking sheet with foil and brush with olive oil.
3. Transfer salmon fillets skin-side down on a baking sheet and spread 1 tablespoon pesto on each fillet.
4. Roast for 20 minutes.
5. Serve and enjoy!

Nutritional Value Per Serving:

Net carbs 1 g

Fiber 2 g

Fats 10 g

Sugar 3 g

Calories 182

Grilled Lemon Shrimps

Prep time: 1 hour

Cook time: 6 minutes

Serves: 3

Difficulty: Intermediate

Ingredients:

- 1 lb. fresh shrimps, cleaned
- 1 tbsp fresh rosemary
- 4 tbsp extra-virgin olive oil
- 1 tsp garlic powder
- 2 tbsp lemon juice, freshly squeezed
- ½ tsp salt
- ½ tsp black pepper, freshly ground
- ½ tsp dried thyme, ground
- ½ tsp dried oregano, ground
- 1 organic lemon, sliced into wedges

Instructions:

1. Combine olive oil, garlic, lemon juice, salt, pepper, thyme, and oregano in a medium bowl and mix until well incorporated. Place the shrimp and coat evenly with the marinade mixture. Cover the bowl and chill for at least 1 hour to marinate the shrimps.

2. Preheat the grill to a medium-high temperature. Brush the grill grids with some oil.

3. Insert 2 to 3 shrimps on each skewer, brush with marinade and grill for 3 minutes. Turn and grill the other side for another 3 minutes. Transfer to a serving platter.

4. Serve warm with lemons wedges and sprinkle with chopped parsley.

Nutritional Value Per Serving:

Net carbs 6.2 g

Fiber 2 g

Fats 21.6 g

Sugar 3 g

Calories 357

Marinated Tuna

Prep time: 2 hours 5 minutes

Cook time: 10 minutes

Serves: 6

Difficulty: Expert

Ingredients:

- 2 lbs. tuna steaks, boneless
- ¼ cup fresh coriander, chopped
- 2 garlic cloves, minced
- 2 tablespoons lemon juice
- 1 cup olive oil
- ½ tsp smoked paprika
- ½ tsp cumin, ground
- ½ tsp chili pepper, ground
- ½ tsp salt
- ¼ tsp black pepper, ground

Instructions:

1. Add the coriander, garlic, paprika, cumin, chili and lemon juice in a food processor and pulse to combine. Gradually add in the oil and mix the ingredients until a smooth mixture.

2. Transfer the mixture into a bowl, add the fish and gently toss to coat the fish evenly with sauce. Chill for at least 2 hours to allow the flavors to penetrate into the fish.

3. Remove the fish from the chiller and preheat the grill. Lightly brush the grid with oil, place the fish on the grid, and grill for about 3 to 4 minutes on each side.

4. Remove the fish from the grill, transfer to a serving plate and serve with lemon wedges or some vegetables.

Nutritional Value Per Serving:

Net carbs 0.7 g

Fiber 1 g

Fats 11.9 g

Sugar 4 g

Calories 303

Broiled White Fish Parmesan

Prep time: 5 minutes

Cook time: 10 minutes

Serves: 4

Difficulty: Expert

Ingredients:

- 3 ounces, Codfish
- ¼ cup, Parmesan cheese, grated
- 2 tablespoons, Light margarine, softened
- 1/8 teaspoon, Garlic salt
- 1/8 teaspoon, Ground black pepper
- 1 tablespoon, Lemon juice
- 1 tablespoon and 1½ teaspoons, Mayonnaise
- 1/8 teaspoon, Dried basil
- 1/8teaspoon, Onion powder
- Cooking spray

Instructions:

1. Set the grill on high temperature and preheat before start cooking.
2. Grease the broiling pot with cooking spray.
3. Combine butter, Parmesan cheese, lemon juice and mayonnaise.
4. Season it with pepper, onion powder, dried basil, and garlic salt.
5. Mix it well and keep ready to use.
6. Layer the fillets on the broiler pan and broil for 2-3 minutes.
7. Flip it and cook for another 2-3 minutes.

8. Remove the baked fillets from the grill onto a plate and transfer the Parmesan mixture over it.

9. Again, broil it for a couple of minutes until the topping becomes brown.

10. Serve hot, when the flakes can easily remove.

Nutritional Value Per Serving:

Net carbs 1 g

Fiber 1 g

Fats 8.2 g

Sugar 2 g

Calories 197.1 g

Grilled Mediterranean Ahi Tuna

Prep time: 15 minutes

Cook time: 10 minutes

Serves: 4

Difficulty: Intermediate

Ingredients:

- 4½ ounces, Ahi tuna steaks, Fresh
- 1 tablespoon, Extra virgin olive oil
- ½ teaspoon Salt
- ½ teaspoon, Lemon juice
- ¼ teaspoon, Cracked black pepper
- ½ teaspoon, Oregano, finely chopped
- ¼ teaspoon, Red pepper, ground
- 1 teaspoon, Basil, finely chopped
- 1 clove Garlic, finely minced

Instructions:

1. Set the charcoal grill on high heat for 30 minutes before you start grilling the tuna steak.
2. Wash and clean the tuna.
3. Pat dry before marinating and put in a shallow bowl.
4. In a small bowl mix all the spices with oil and lemon juice.
5. Allow the mixture to have a rest for 5 minutes so that everything blends well. If you are sensitive to spices, use a fork/spoon to mix the spices.
6. Now, marinate the tuna steaks applying the mixture with a brush.
7. Allow it to settle for 5 minutes.

8. Grill all the steaks on a hot grill at least for 3-5 minutes for both sides to get the desired result.

9. When the fish grilled well, it will turn to pinkish at the center.

10. Don't overcook.

Nutritional Value Per Serving:

Net carbs 0.5 g

Fiber 0.1 g

Fats 5.3 g

Sugar 4 g

Calories 229.2

Herb-Crusted Salmon Fillets

Prep time: 10 minutes

Cook time: 10 minutes

Serves: 4

Difficulty: Expert

Ingredients

- 16 ounces, Atlantic salmon
- 2 tablespoons, Chives, roughly chopped
- 2 tablespoons, Parsley, chopped
- 1 cup, Breadcrumbs, whole-grain
- ½ teaspoon, Garlic powder
- ½ teaspoon, Onion powder
- 1 teaspoon, Lemon peel, grated
- ¼ cup, Lemon juice
- ¼ teaspoon, Salt
- ½ teaspoon, Pepper
- Cooking spray.

Instructions

1. Preheat the oven on high heat at 400°F.
2. Line the baking tray with a baking paper and spray some cooking oil.
3. Season the salmon fillets with pepper and salt.
4. Place the salmon on the baking tray, skin side down facing the baking liner.

5. Put all the ingredients except lemon juice in mixer bowl.

6. Combine well until it becomes a smooth mix.

7. Drizzle some lemon juice on the salmon fillets and spread the breadcrumb mixture over the salmon fillets.

8. Spray evenly with cooking spray, and bake it at least for 10 - 15 minutes.

9. Serve hot.

Nutritional Value Per Serving:

Net carbs 7.2 g

Fiber 1.1 g

Fats 14.4 g

Sugar 2 g

Calories 259.5

Honey and Soy Glazed Salmon

Prep time: 10 minutes

Cook time: 7 minutes

Serves: 2

Difficulty: Beginner

Ingredients:

- 2 filets, Salmon
- 2 tablespoons, Honey
- 1½ tablespoons, Lime juice
- 2 tablespoons, Soy sauce, low sodium
- 2 tablespoons, Vegetable oil
- 2 teaspoons, Mustard
- 1 tablespoon, Water

Instructions

1. In a medium bowl, whisk honey, soy sauce, mustard, lime juice, and water.
2. Pour vegetable oil into a non-stick skillet and bring to high heat.
3. Roast the filets at least for 2 to 3 minutes and flip sides and continue roasting for another 2-3 minutes, until it becomes brown.
4. Transfer filets into a serving plate.
5. Add some honey glaze to the skillet and heat for one minute.
6. Pour the honey glaze over salmon and serve hot.

Nutritional Value Per Serving:

Net carbs 21.3 g

Fiber 0.7 g

Fats 11.2 g

Sugar 2 g

Calories 277.3 g

Lemon Garlic Tilapia

Prep time: 5 minutes

Cook time: 30 minutes

Serves: 4

Difficulty: Intermediate

Ingredients:

- 4 fillets, Tilapia

- 1 tablespoon, Olive oil

- 1 tablespoon, Margarine

- 1 tablespoon, Lemon juice

- ¼ teaspoon, Salt

- 1 teaspoon, Garlic salt

- 1 teaspoon, Parsley flakes, dried

- ¼ teaspoon, Cayenne pepper

- Cooking spray

Instructions:

1. Set the temperature of the oven at 400°F and start preheating.

2. Spray nonstick cooking oil onto the baking tray.

3. Put the butter into a nonstick saucepan and melt it on low-medium heat.

4. Now, add some lemon juice, salt, olive oil, garlic powder, and parsley into it and sauté for 3-4 minutes.

5. Place the tilapia fillets in the baking tray and pour the preparation on the top of the fillets.

6. Now sprinkle some cayenne pepper on the fish.

7. Put in the oven and bake for about 12-13 minutes.

8. Flip sides and cook it for extra time.

9. Serve hot

Nutritional Value Per Serving:

Net carbs 1.8 g

Fiber 0.3 g

Fats 7.3 g

Sugar 3 g

Calories 175.2

Lime Shrimp

Prep time: 3 minutes

Cook time: 10 minutes

Serves: 2

Ingredients

- 28 Shrimps, ready to cook
- 1 tablespoon, Lime juice
- 1/8 teaspoon, Salt
- ¾ teaspoon, Black pepper
- 2 tablespoons, Chopped onion
- Cooking spray

Instructions:

1. Spray some cooking oil into the skillet.
2. Bring the skillet to medium heat.
3. When the skillet becomes hot, put all the ingredients and sauté occasionally until the onions and shrimps get cooked well.
4. Serve hot

Nutritional Value Per Serving:

Net carbs 2.2 g

Fiber 0.4 g

Fats 0.9 g

Sugar 1 g

Calories 84.4

Microwave Grilled Salmon

Prep time: 5 minutes

Cook time: 4 minutes

Serves: 4

Difficulty: Beginner

Ingredients:

- 1½ pound, Salmon
- 2 tablespoons, Olive oil
- 1 tablespoon, Lemon juice
- 1 clove, Garlic, minced
- ¼ teaspoon, Salt
- ¼ teaspoon, Ground pepper

Instructions:

1. Set your microwave to grill cooking.
2. In a medium bowl, mix all the ingredients.
3. Marinate the salmon.
4. Grill the fish.
5. Serve hot.

Nutritional Value Per Serving:

Net carbs 0.4 g

Fiber 1 g

Fats 9.5 g

Sugar 2 g

Calories 210.2

Tuna Salad

Prep time: 10 minutes

Serves: 4

Difficulty: Beginner

Ingredients:

- 2 pounds, Tuna cooked
- 1 stalk, Celery, finely chopped
- 2/3 cup, Cottage cheese, non-fat
- 4 tablespoons, Plain yogurt, low-fat
- ¼, Small onion, red, coarsely chopped
- 1 teaspoon, Dijon mustard
- 1 teaspoon, Lemon juice
- ¼ teaspoon, Dill
- ½ teaspoon, Salt

Instructions:

1. In a large bowl, mix all the ingredients to make the salad.
2. Ideal for making sandwiches.

Nutritional Value Per Serving:

Net carbs 11.7 g

Fiber 0.6 g

Fats 2.2 g

Sugar 1 g

Calories 190.3

Vegan recipes
Chickpea Curry

Prep time: 10 minutes

Cook time: 20 minutes

Serves: 4

Difficulty: Expert

Ingredients

- 1 can Chickpeas
- 1 tablespoon Olive oil
- 1 Large onion, chopped
- 1½ tablespoon, Ginger powder
- 1 tablespoon, Cumin
- ½ tablespoon Salt
- 1/8 tablespoon Black pepper, crushed
- 5 cloves Garlic, minced
- 5 tablespoons, Curry powder
- 1 Tomato, large and chopped
- 1/8 teaspoon, Cinnamon
- 1/8 teaspoon, Oregano
- 2/3 cup, Water

Instructions:

1. Rinse and drain the chickpeas.
2. Pour olive oil in a large nonstick cooking pan and bring to low-medium heat.
3. When the oil becomes hot, put the onion and sauté.

4. Continue sautéing for about 4-5 minutes, until the onion becomes translucent.

5. Add garlic and cook for about 1 min.

6. Now add ginger and curry powder in into the pan.

7. Stir to mix thoroughly and cook for about 1 more minute.

8. Now add chickpeas, cumin, salt, pepper, cinnamon, and water to the pan.

9. Stir to mix well.

10. Continue cooking by adding tomato and herbs of oregano.

11. Stir occasionally and cook for a couple of minutes.

12. Cover the pan and cook on low heat until the tomatoes become soft.

13. Stir intermittently to avoid sticking.

14. After the tomatoes become soft, open the lid and check the sausage consistency. If you wish to reduce the sauce, continue heating for a few minutes more.

15. Serve hot.

Nutritional Value Per Serving:

Net carbs 29.0 g

Fiber 6.2 g

Fats 5.0 g

Sugar 3 g

Calories 177.3

Blue Oatmeal Porridge

Prep time: 2 minutes

Cook time: 5 minutes

Serves: 2

Difficulty: Beginner

Ingredients:

- 1 cup, Whole grain oatmeal
- 2 tablespoons, Flaxseed meal, ground flax
- ½ tablespoon, Dry cocoa powder, unsweetened
- 2 teaspoon, Brown sugar
- ½ cup, Blueberries, frozen, unsweetened
- 1½ cup, Water

Instructions:

1. Boil water in a pan.
2. Combine all of the dry ingredients in a mixing bowl and add to the boiling water.
3. Reduce the temperature and cook it for a couple of minutes as far as you get the desired consistency.
4. Top it with blueberries at the time of serving.

Nutritional Value Per Serving:

Net carbs 38.4 g

Fiber 7 g

Fats 5.7 g

Sugar 1 g

Calories 214.2

Garlic and Olive Oil Spaghetti Squash

Prep time: 5 minutes

Cook time: 1 hour

Serves: 2

Difficulty: Intermediate

Ingredients:

- 1 Spaghetti squash
- 2 tablespoons, Olive oil
- 3 cloves Garlic, minced
- ¼ cup Water
- ¼ teaspoon, Pepper crushed
- ¼ teaspoon, Salt

Instructions:

1. Cut the squash in lengthwise into two parts.
2. Scoop out all the seeds, and save the seeds.
3. In a casserole place the squash, face down and pour a quarter cup of water.
4. Bake the squash at 375°F temperature for 30 minutes.
5. Flip the squash to cook the other side for an extra 30 minutes until it becomes soft.
6. Allow squash to settle down.
7. Now, in a sauté pan pour olive oil and bring to low-medium heat.
8. When the oil becomes hot add garlic and sauté.
9. With the use of a serving fork, transfer the boiled squash into the sautéing pan.
10. Add some salt and pepper
11. Cook it for 3-5 minutes more.

12. Serve hot.

Nutritional Value Per Serving:

Net carbs 14.5 g

Fiber 2.9 g

Fats 14.5 g

Sugar 4 g

Calories 181.4

Grilled Cheese Pizza Sandwich

Prep time: 2 minutes

Cook time: 5 minutes

Serves: 1

Difficulty: Beginner

Ingredients:

- 2 slices, Multi-grain bread
- 2 tablespoons, Marinara sauce
- 1 teaspoon, Shredded Parmesan
- ¼ cup, Mozzarella cheese
- ¼ teaspoon, Pepper ground
- ¼ teaspoon, Salt

Instructions:

1. Spread the marinara sauce on one side of both bread slice.
2. Now spread mozzarella cheese on top of one slice bread.
3. Sprinkle grated Parmesan cheese on the top of the mozzarella.
4. Top it with 2nd piece of bread, keeping the sauce side down.
5. Now place it on a heated pan until the cheese starts to melt and the outer side becomes golden brown.
6. Serve hot.

Nutritional Value Per Serving:

Net carbs 26.3 g

Fiber 4.4 g

Fats 8.3 g

Sugar 6 g

Calories 242.3

Mini Eggplant Pizzas

Prep time: 5 minutes

Cook time: 12 minutes

Serves: 4

Difficulty: Intermediate

Ingredients:

- 1 Eggplant
- ¼ cup, Pasta sauce
- 4 teaspoons, Olive oil
- ½ teaspoon, Salt

- 1/8 teaspoon, Ground black pepper
- ½ cup, Shredded part-skim mozzarella cheese
- Cooking spray
- Baking sheet

Instructions:

1. Peel eggplant and cut into 4 half-inch-thick slices.
2. Preheat your toaster at 425°F.
3. Brush both parts of the eggplant with some cooking spray oil and season it with pepper and salt.
4. Arrange the pizza on a baking sheet and bake for 8 minutes, until it becomes browned and tender.
5. Flip sides and bake further 6 - 8 minutes.
6. Spread 1 tbsp of pasta sauce on all side of the sliced eggplant.
7. Top it with the shredded cheese.
8. Bake the cheese until it starts to melt for about 3 - 5 minutes.
9. Serve the dish hot.

Nutritional Value Per Serving:

Net carbs 8.9 g

Fiber 3.2 g

Fats 7.5 g

Sugar 8 g

Calories 119.1

131

Oven-Roasted Brussels Sprouts

Prep time: 5 minutes

Cook time: 30 minutes

Serves: 4

Difficulty: Beginner

Ingredients:

- 15 to 20, Fresh Brussels Sprouts
- Non-fat spray for cooking
- 2 tablespoons, Olive oil
- ½ teaspoon, Ground black pepper
- ¼ teaspoon, Salt

Instructions:

1. Set your oven at 425°F and put it on for preheating.
2. Trim all the stems from sprouts.
3. Cut sprouts in lengthwise into wo equal parts.
4. Take a shallow baking dish and spray with cooking oil.
5. Place all the sprouts in the center of dish keep the cut-side up.
6. Drizzle olive oil on top of it.
7. Similarly, drizzle salt and ground pepper.
8. Bake it for 15 minutes, and flip sides after ten minutes.
9. Serve hot with fresh tomato soup or parmesan zucchini.

Nutritional Value Per Serving:

Net carbs 6.7 g

Fiber 2.8 g

Fats 3.6 g

Sugar 2 g

Calories 61.8

Portobello Mushrooms Bake

Prep time: 10 minutes

Cook time: 25 minutes

Serves: 4

Difficulty: Intermediate

Ingredients:

- 3 caps, Portabella mushroom, large
- 2 cups, Instant brown rice
- 1 cup, Black bans
- 1 cup, Red pepper pieces

- 2 tablespoons, Olive oil
- 3 ounces, Shredded mozzarella, part-skim
- ¼ teaspoon, Garlic, minced
- ¼ teaspoon, Salt

Instructions:

1. In a medium saucepan pour olive oil and sauté red pepper and garlic until it becomes soft.
2. Add the mushrooms and continue sautéing for 5 minutes.
3. After cooking, stop heating and remove from the pan.
4. Now boil rice as per the given instructions in the packet.
5. Mix the rice with black beans in a casserole dish.
6. Add the mushroom caps in the rice and black bean mix.
7. Make the topping with roasted red peppers and mozzarella cheese.
8. Bake at 350°F temperature for 18-20 minutes until cheese becomes bubbly.

Nutritional Value Per Serving:

Net carbs 39 g

Fiber 7.1 g

Fats 10.5 g

Sugar 5 g

Calories 288.8

Spaghetti Squash Marinara

Prep time: 5 minutes

Cook time: 50 minutes

Serves: 2

Difficulty: Intermediate

Ingredients:

- 1 Raw spaghetti squash, medium
- 14 ½ ounces Stewed tomatoes, cut up, canned
- 1 teaspoon, Italian seasoning
- 1 teaspoon, Olive oil
- 1, Small onion, chopped
- 1 teaspoon, Garlic clove, minced
- ¼ cup, Parmesan cheese, grated

Instructions

1. Set the oven at 350°F and start preheating.
2. Cut the squash lengthwise into two equal parts and scoop out all the seeds.
3. Place all the squash, in a large baking dish keeping the cut sides down and pierce the skin with a fork.
4. Bake it until it becomes soft for about 30 - 40 minutes.
5. Now let us make the sauce.
6. Heat some oil in a small skillet on medium temperature.
7. Add garlic, onion and sauté about 5 minutes, until it becomes tender.
8. Add Italian seasoning, tomatoes and bring to boil.
9. Reduce the heat and continue cooking for about 5 minutes, without covering the skillet, until you get the desired consistency.

10. Now before serving, carefully take out the squash pulp in strands with a fork, as if looks like spaghetti.

11. Pour sauce on the top of the squash and sprinkle some Parmesan cheese on top.

Nutritional Value Per Serving:

Net carbs 12.4 g

Fiber 2.1 g

Fats 3.3 g

Sugar 1 g

Calories 88.6

Vegan Lentil Burgers

Prep time: 10 minutes

Cook time: 1 hour

Serves: 8

Difficulty: Expert

Ingredients

- 1 cup, Brown rice, uncooked
- 1 cup, Lentils, uncooked
- 1½ cup, Carrots, finely grated
- 1½ cup, Oatmeal, uncooked
- ½ teaspoon, Garlic powder
- 1 teaspoon, Salt
- 1 Small onion, coarsely chopped
- 4 cups, Water
- Cooking spray

Instructions

1. In a large bowl pour four cups of water and cook the rice and the lentils, at low heat for 45 minutes by keeping the lid closed.

2. After cooking, allow it to settle and cool.

3. Add all the remaining ingredients gradually and mix well.

4. Mold into patties

5. Spray some cooking oil and bring to low heart.

6. When the pan becomes hot, place the patties and cook for 6 minutes until it becomes brown.

7. Flip sides and cook another 6 minutes.

8. Use as a burger with your favorite sauce.

Nutritional Value Per Serving:

Net carbs 24.2 g	Fats 1.5 g	Calories 127.6
Fiber 4.8 g	Sugar 5 g	

Desserts

Strawberry Frozen Yogurt Squares

Prep time: 8 hours

Serves: 8

Difficulty: Beginner

Ingredients:

- 1 cup barley, wheat cereal
- 3 cup fat-free strawberry yogurt
- 10 oz. frozen strawberries
- 1 cup fat- free milk
- 1 cup whipped topping

Instructions:

1. Set a parchment paper on the baking tray.
2. Spread cereal evenly over the bottom of the tray.
3. Add milk, strawberries and yogurt to blender, and process into a smooth mixture.
4. Use yogurt mixture to top cereal, wrap with foil, and place to freeze until firm (about 8 hours).
5. Slightly thaw, slice into squares and serve.

Nutritional Value Per Serving:

Net carbs 43.4 g

Fiber 4 g

Fats 3 g

Sugar 7 g

Calories 188

Smoked Tofu Quesadillas

Prep time: 6 minutes

Cook time: 5 minutes

Serves: 4

Difficulty: Beginner

Ingredients:

- 1 lb. extra firm sliced tofu

- 12 tortillas

- 2 tbsps. coconut oil

- 6 slices cheddar cheese

- 2 tbsps. sundried tomatoes

- 1 tbsp. cilantro

- 5 tbsps. sour cream

Instructions:

1. Lay one tortilla flat and fill with tofu, tomato, cheese and top with oil. Repeat for as many as you need.

2. Bake for 5 minutes and remove from flame.

3. Top with sour cream.

Nutritional Value Per Serving:

Net carbs 13 g

Fiber 3 g

Fats 6 g

Sugar 3 g

Calories 136

Zucchini Pizza Boats

Prep time: 5 minutes

Cook time: 30 minutes

Serves: 2

Difficulty: Beginner

Ingredients:

- 2 medium Zucchini
- ½ cup Tomato Sauce
- ½ cup shredded Mozzarella cheese
- 2 tbsps. Parmesan cheese

Instructions:

1. Set oven to 350 degrees F.
2. Slice zucchini in half lengthwise and spoon out the core and seeds to form boats.
3. Place zucchini halves skin side down in a small baking dish.
4. Add remaining ingredients inside the hollow center then set to bake until golden brown and fork tender (about 30 minutes).
5. Serve and enjoy.

Nutritional Value Per Serving:

Net carbs 23.6 g

Fiber 4 g

Fats 7.9 g

Sugar 1 g

Calories 214

Pear-Cranberry Pie with Oatmeal Streusel

Prep time: 10 minutes

Cook time: 1 hour

Serves: 6

Difficulty: Intermediate

Ingredients:

Streusel:

- ¾ cup oats
- 1/3 cup stevia
- ½ tsp. cinnamon
- ¼ tsp. nutmeg
- 1 tbsp. cubed butter

Filling:

- 3 cup cubed pears
- 2 cup cranberries
- ½ cup stevia
- 2½ tbsps. cornstarch

Instructions:

1. Set oven to 350 degrees F.
2. Combine all streusel ingredients in a food processor and process into a coarse crumb.
3. Next, combine all filling ingredients in a large bowl and toss to combine.
4. Transfer filling into pie crust, then top with streusel mix.
5. Set to bake until golden brown (about an hour). Cool and serve.

Nutritional Value Per Serving:

Net carbs 47 g

Fiber 4 g

Fats 9 g

Sugar 1 g

Calories 280

Macerated Summer Berries with Frozen Yogurt

Prep time: 2 hours

Serves: 4

Difficulty: Beginner

Ingredients:

- 1 cup sliced strawberries
- 1 cup blueberries
- 1 cup raspberries
- 1 tbsp. stevia
- 1 tsp. orange zest
- 2 tbsps. orange juice
- 1 pint low fat yogurt

Instructions:

1. Add stevia, orange zest, orange juice and berries to a large bowl.
2. Toss to combine. Set to chill for at least 2 hours.
3. Divide yogurt evenly into 4 serving bowls, top evenly with berry mixture and serve.

Nutritional Value Per Serving:

Net carbs 28.4 g

Fiber 10 g

Fats 1 g

Sugar 2 g

Calories 133

Pumpkin Pie Spiced Yogurt

Prep time: 15 minutes

Serves: 2

Difficulty: Beginner

Ingredients:

- 2 cup low fat plain yogurt
- ½ cup pumpkin puree
- ¼ tsp. cinnamon
- ¼ tsp. pumpkin pie spice
- ¼ cup chopped walnuts
- 1 tbsp. honey

Instructions:

1. Combine spices with the pumpkin puree in a medium bowl and stir.
2. Stir in yogurt, divide into 2 serving glasses. Top with honey and walnuts. Serve and enjoy!

Nutritional Value Per Serving:

Net carbs 22 g

Fiber 1 g

Fats 7 g

Sugar 10 g

Calories 208

Tropical Dreams Pudding

Prep time: 10 minutes

Serves: 4

Difficulty: Beginner

Ingredients:

- 1 package sugar-free fat-free banana instant pudding mix

- 2 cups cold skim milk

- 4 scoops tropical fruit-flavored low-carb whey protein isolate powder

Instructions:

1. In a medium bowl, beat pudding mix, milk and protein powder with an electric hand mixer until thoroughly blended and slightly thickened, about 2 minutes.

2. Pour pudding into 4 small bowls and refrigerate until set, about 5 minutes. Serve immediately, or cover and refrigerate for up to 2 days. Enjoy!

Nutritional Value Per Serving:

Net carbs 12 g

Fiber 1 g

Fats 10 g

Sugar 2 g

Calories 125

Green Tea Smoothie

Prep time: 10 minutes

Serves: 2

Difficulty: Intermediate

Ingredients:

- 3 tbsp green tea powder
- 1 cup grapes, white
- ½ cup kale, finely chopped
- 1 tbsp honey
- ½ tsp fresh mint, ground
- 1 cup water

Instructions:

1. Rinse the grapes under cold running water. Drain and remove the pits. Set aside.

2. Place kale in a large colander and wash thoroughly under cold running water. Drain well and finely chop it into small pieces. Set aside.

3. Combine green tea powder with 2 tablespoons of hot water. Soak for 2 minutes. Set aside.

4. Now, combine grapes, kale, honey, mint, and water in a blender and process until well combined. Stir in the water and tea mixture.

5. Refrigerate 30 minutes before serving.

6. Enjoy!

Nutritional Value Per Serving:

Net carbs 18.3 g

Fiber 2.2 g

Fats 0.2 g

Sugar 1 g

Calories 76

Conclusion

I sincerely hope that the book has succeeded in its aim to educate you about gastric sleeve surgery and the associated diet plan. The recipes contained in this book will help you in your recovery process.

To engage in the process, consult your doctor to ensure that you are physically fit and psychologically prepared. It should have been informative and provided you with all of the tools needed to achieve your goals, whatever they may be.

The next step is to talk to your doctor if you feel a gastric sleeve surgery is for you. If you already have one scheduled, you are ready to start trying out the recipes. This book will be there for you before, during, and after your surgery. The important thing is to make sure you are prepared.

CPSIA information can be obtained
at www.ICGtesting.com
Printed in the USA
LVHW100804231020
669519LV00001B/72